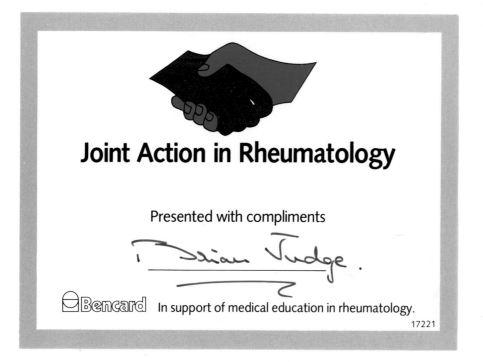

Joint Action in Rheumatology

Presented with compliments

Brian Judge.

Bencard In support of medical education in rheumatology.

17221

An Atlas of
Radiology of Rheumatic Disorders

Prof. Dr. J. Dequeker
M.D., PhD., F.R.C.P. (Edin.)
Rheumatology Section
Department of Internal Medicine
Akademische Ziekenhuizen
Katholieke Universiteit
Leuven, Belgium

English version by D.H. Bosman, M.B., Ch.B., M.Sc.,
Royal College of Surgeons of England.

Wolfe Medical Publications Ltd

General Editor, Wolfe Medical Atlases:
G. Barry Carruthers, MD(Lond)

Copyright © J. Dequeker, 1982
Published by Wolfe Medical Publications Ltd, 1982
Printed by Royal Smeets Offset b.v., Weert, Netherlands
ISBN 0 7234 0773 8

This book is one of the titles in the series of
Wolfe Medical Atlases, a series which brings
together probably the world's largest systematic
published collection of diagnostic colour
photographs.
For a full list of Atlases in the series, plus
forthcoming titles and details of our surgical,
dental and veterinary Atlases, please write to
Wolfe Medical Publications Ltd, Wolfe House,
3 Conway Street, London W1P 6HE

Contents

Preface

My interest in the radiology of rheumatic diseases has been greatly influenced on the one hand by Professor S. de Sèze (Paris), who taught me how to analyse in detail skeletal X-rays and correlate them with clinical data, and on the other hand by the work of Dr. A. Ryckewaert (Paris) and Dr. W. Dihlmann (Hamburg), who elucidated the principle of explanatory line drawings.

The correct interpretation of a bone X-ray does not depend so much on the quality of the X-ray picture as on a knowledge of the patient's clinical data and a full understanding of the anatomy and pathophysiology of bone and joint diseases. Although the radiographic signs come relatively late in the course of rheumatic diseases, radiology can be of considerable help in confirming a clinical diagnosis, especially when typical lesions are seen.

It should not be the pathognomonic lesion of the final stage of rheumatic disease which is sought, but the earliest changes in detail. It is therefore necessary to examine X-rays very closely – with a magnifying glass in those areas where the clinical manifestations are most prominent.

This book is designed in such a way that the reader becomes involved in making a diagnosis. A short summary of the case accompanies the radiograph concerned. A drawing of the radiographic lesions indicates the areas to which particular attention should be given. A diagnosis, together with the description of discoverable lesions, is followed by a brief discussion.

The aim is not to give an encyclopaedic survey of all the possible processes affecting the skeleton but to indicate the variety of diagnoses that rheumatic complaints or abnormalities can present in the bones and joints. An accurate diagnosis should point to correct treatment, which does not consist only of antirheumatic agents.

Acknowledgements

I am grateful to my colleagues in the Department of Internal Medicine and Orthopaedics for their referral of some patients illustrated here and to the doctors of the Department of Radiology for assisting at the weekly clinico-radiology meeting at the Rheumatology unit.

The Atlas could not have been compiled without the generous help of Parke-Davis Belgium, who stimulated me to bring together this collection, of Mr. A. Rummens for photographic assistance and of Mrs. J. Cartois for secretarial help.

: Hand and elbow

though skeletal structures lend themselves readily to
iographic examination, and gross changes present
ical pictures, the usefulness of radiography in the
rly stages proves rather limited. In the majority of
umatic affections however, after a certain degree of
velopment, specific lesions come to the fore which
helpful in differential diagnosis.

Since anatomical differences frequently occur, it is
cessary to obtain pictures of both left and right joints
comparison even when only one joint is affected.
e radiographs should always be examined closely,
ing a magnifying glass and a strong light. The lesions,
ch as incipient erosion and periosteal reaction, can be
ry faint. In assessing altered translucency, say for
ample a periarticular osteoporosis, the presence of
erlying synovial thickening must be borne in mind.

The radiograph of a hand can be useful in the diagno-
of a process involving the hand itself but may also aid
diagnosing a more generalised condition where the
tient may experience no hand symptoms.

1

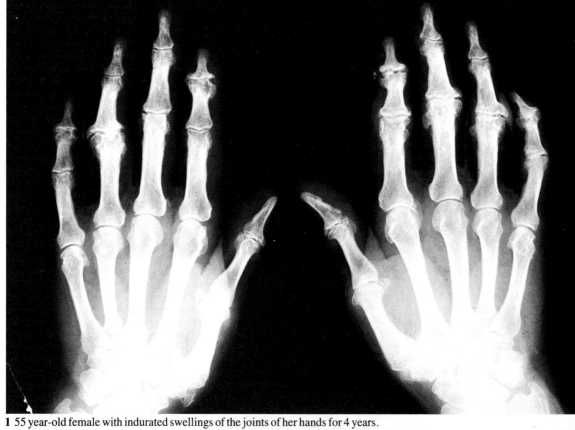

1 55 year-old female with indurated swellings of the joints of her hands for 4 years.

2

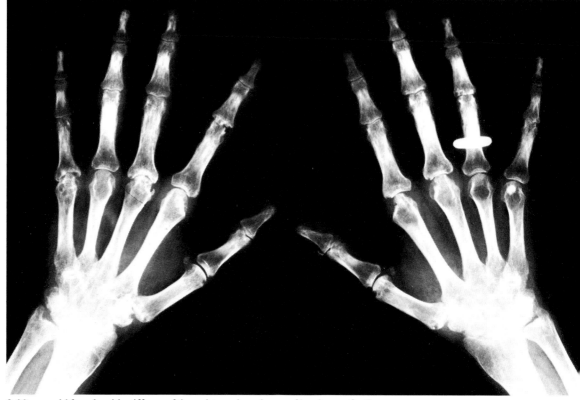

2 30 year-old female with stiffness of the wrists and weakness of her fingers for 7 years.

Polyarthrosis

generative lesions in the region of the small
nts of the hand: irregular narrowing of the joint
ces, subchondral sclerosis, osteophytosis.
berden's nodes (1), Bouchard's nodes (2),
hropathy of the root of the thumb (rhizarthro-
) (3), cystic translucency (4).

e abnormalities in the region of the distal joints
st not be confused with those of psoriatic
hropathy.
ur grades of arthropathy are distinguished:
ade 1: normal joint apart from minimal
:eophyte formation;
ade 2: visible osteophytosis at two points with
nimal subchondral sclerosis, good joint space,
malformation;
ade 3: moderate osteophytosis, ensuing mal-
rmation of ends of bone, narrowing of the joint
ace;
ade 4: large osteophyte, malformation of the
ne ends, narrowed joint space, sclerosis and
st formation.

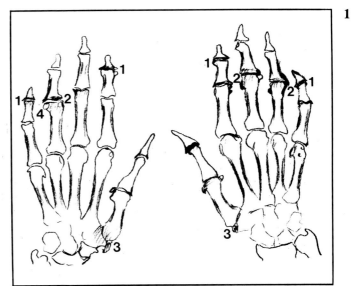

1

Rheumatoid arthritis: Stage IV

riarticular osteoporosis (1), uniform narrow-
g of joint spaces (2), erosions (3), ankylosis (4).
e sharp, sclerotic outline of the erosions indi-
tes inactive arthritis.

ur radiological stages of rheumatoid arthritis
e distinguished:
age 1: normal bone, periarticular osteoporosis,
ft tissue swelling;
age 2: slight narrowing of the joint space;
age 3: cartilage and bone destruction;
age 4: fibrous or bony ankylosis.

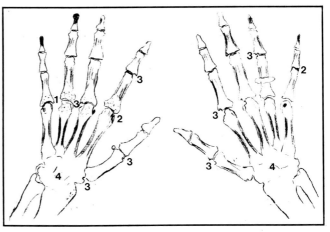

2

3

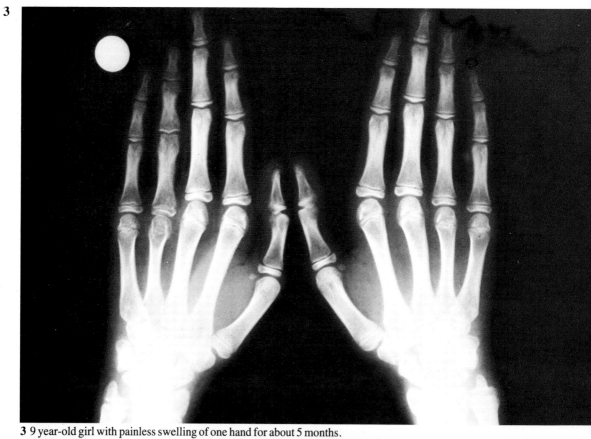

3 9 year-old girl with painless swelling of one hand for about 5 months.

4

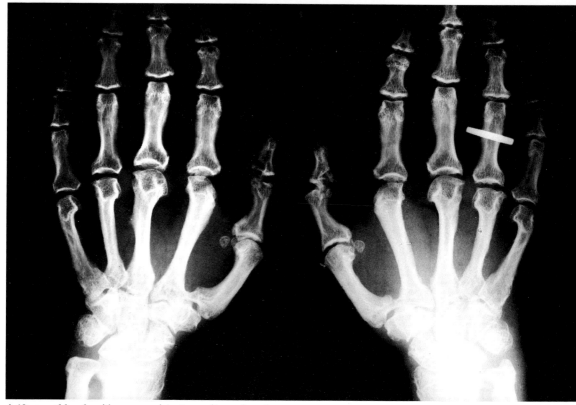

4 40 year-old male with a very resistant carpal tunnel syndrome.

3 Juvenile rheumatoid arthritis

Arthritis of fourth metacarpophalangeal joint on the left side (arrow), periarticular osteoporosis, uniform narrowing of joint space, shortening of the fourth metacarpal due to early closure of growing epiphysis.

Rheumatoid arthritis in children is usually monoarticular and arouses little complaint. Radiologically one needs to note changes around the epiphyses and consequent effects on the growth of the bone concerned which may initially undergo accelerated growth and eventually be shorter due to early closure of the growing epiphysis.

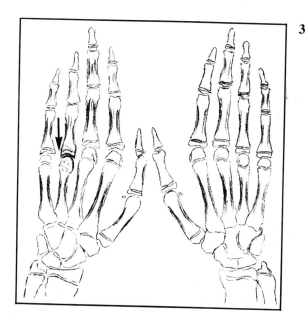

3

4 Acromegaly

Widened articular space due to thickened cartilage (1), bone expansion (periostosis) (2), osteophytosis (3), cystic rarefaction (4).

Untreated acromegaly gives rise to secondary osteoarthropathy due to disintegration of the joint. Besides the bony abnormalities, there is generalised soft tissue swelling which leads to carpal tunnel syndrome amongst other things.

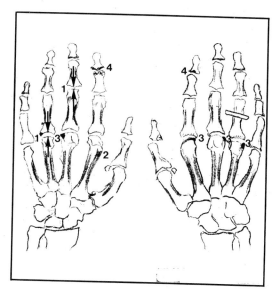

4

5

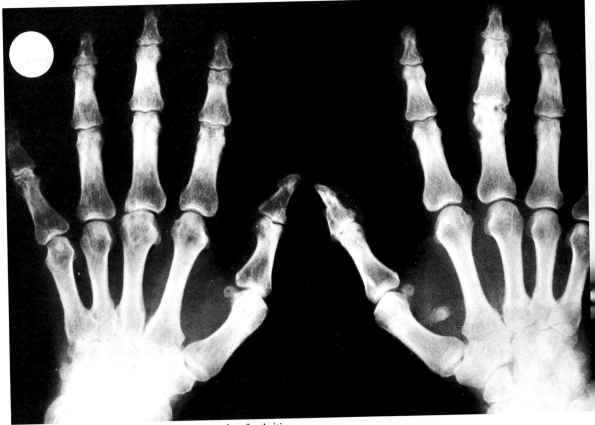

5 55 year-old male with a history of severe attacks of arthritis.

6

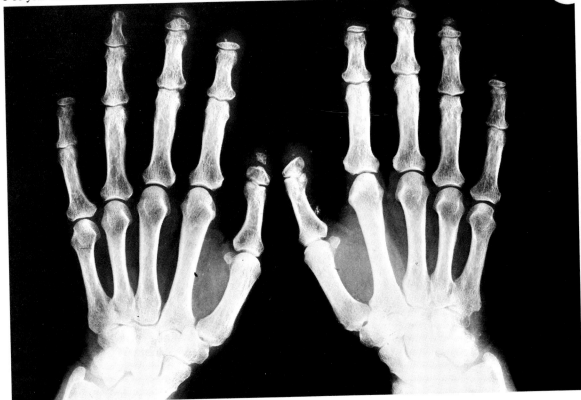

6 77 year-old female with a history of Raynaud's phenomenon for 40 years.

Gouty Arthritis

gular narrowing of the joint space (1), sub-
ndral sclerosis (2), translucencies produced
geodes (3), hypertrophic bone reaction (4),
ylosis of the carpus (5).

arthritis of gout is distinguished from arthro-
y by the presence of bone destruction
des) usually localised at the margin of the
anx some distance from the joint, and by an
ggerated sclerotic reaction.
arthritis is asymmetrical and oligoarticular in
trast to rheumatoid arthritis where symmetri-
oints especially are affected.

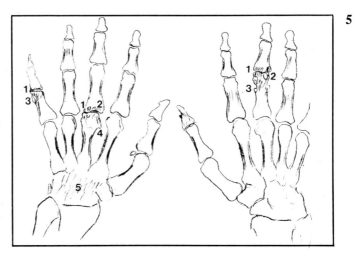

5

Scleroderma

oosteolysis: resorption of the distal pha-
ges.

patient suffered additional disorders of the
phagus, lungs and heart. In scleroderma the
y radiological abnormality is usually frag-
ntation of the distal phalanges.
oosteolysis also occurs in:
rare familial disease with multiple bone abnor-
alities (dysplasias) and osteoporosis (familial
croosteolysis)
heumatoid arthritis (very rarely)
yperparathyroidism
achydermoperiostosis
PVC (polyvinylchloride) workers in the plas-
ics industry
yknodysostosis
Rothmund's syndrome (heredofamilial
atrophic dermatosis)
seudoxanthoma.

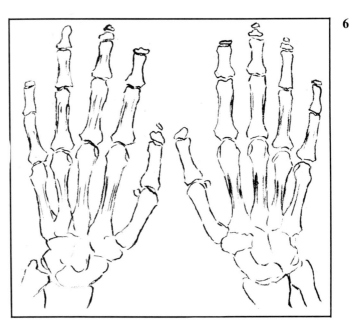

6

7

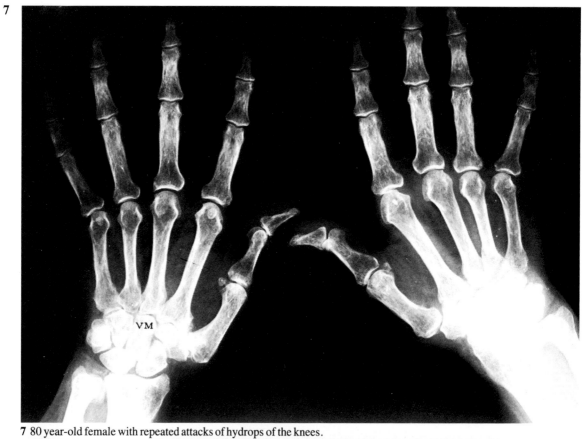

7 80 year-old female with repeated attacks of hydrops of the knees.

8

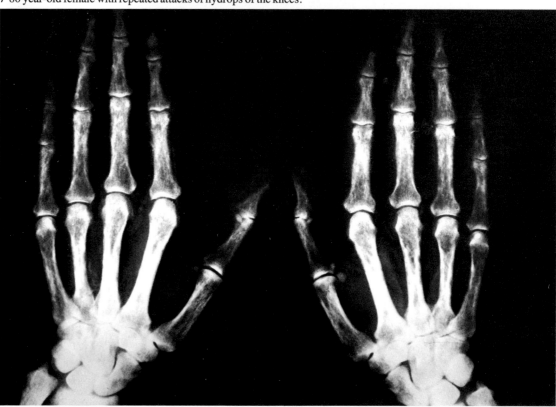

8 40 year-old female under chronic haemodialysis.

Chondrocalcinosis

...cification of the cartilage at the lower end of ...right ulna (1), ulnar osteophytosis at the ...oulnar joint (2), narrowing of the joint space ...he radiocarpal joint with sclerotic reaction (3), ...cortex of metacarpals with widened medul-...cavities (4).

...ondrocalcinosis can present joint symptoms ...embling gout, hence the name pseudogout or ...stal synovitis, due to pyrophosphate crystals. ...ondrocalcinosis can be idiopathic but may also ...associated with other abnormalities which ...e to be excluded: haemochromatosis (in-...ased serum iron), hyperparathyroidism (in-...ased serum calcium), gout (increased serum ...c acid), diabetes mellitus (increased serum ...cose), acromegaly (growth hormone), Wil-...'s disease (increased serum copper).

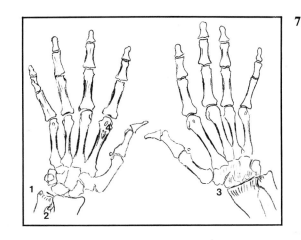

7

Secondary hyperparathyroidism

...gular and poorly outlined bone structure with ...periosteal bone resorption (1), periarticular ...cification (2), arterial calcification (3), ...eolysis of the terminal phalanges (4).

...nal osteodystrophy is the result of various ...hophysiological mechanisms.

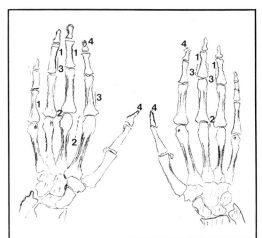

8

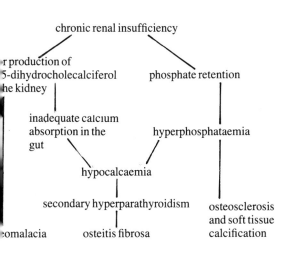

chronic renal insufficiency

...r production of
...5-dihydrocholecalciferol   phosphate retention
...he kidney

inadequate calcium
absorption in the   hyperphosphataemia
gut

hypocalcaemia

secondary hyperparathyroidism   osteosclerosis
                                       and soft tissue
...omalacia   osteitis fibrosa   calcification

9

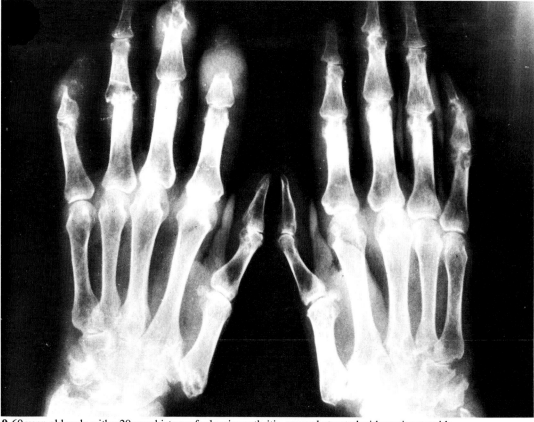

9 60 year-old male with a 20 year history of relapsing arthritis, wrongly treated with corticosteroids.

10

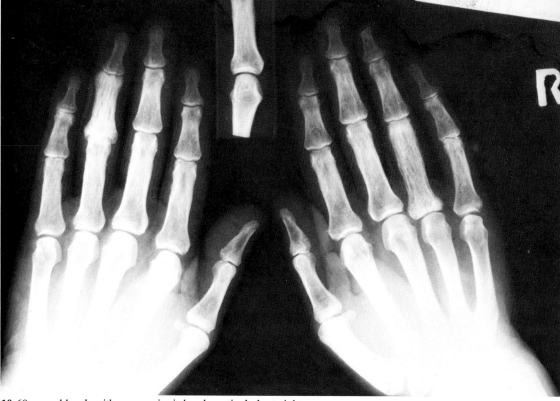

10 60 year-old male with vague pains in hands particularly at night.

Gouty arthritis with tophi

estructive arthritis with significant bone resorp-
on in the vicinity of tophi (1), joint space nar-
wing with bone sclerosis (2), multiple geodes
), subluxation of the trapeziometacarpal joints
), ankylosis and destruction of the carpal bones
).

nal outcome of a wrongly treated gout sufferer.
spite of the enormous joint destruction, the
tient has little pain and only slight disability.
ith well controlled treatment, uricosuric or uric
id synthesis-retarding medication, the tophus
rmation can be prevented. Existing tophi may
sappear completely after some years of treat-
ent.

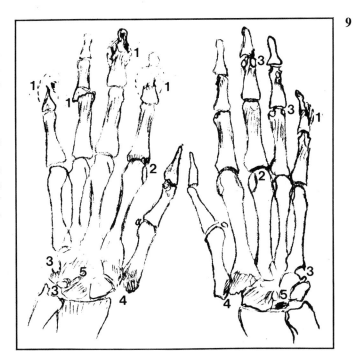

9

) Paget's disease

getoid bony changes in proximal phalanx of
ght ring finger and middle phalanx of left ring
ger (arrow).

ne changes of Paget's disease are characterised
thickening and irregular structure with areas of
lerosis and osteolysis unevenly distributed.
e disease may be monostotic or polyostotic.
ring the active phase the alkaline phosphatase
tivity is high to very high, as is also the hyd-
xyprolinuria. Prolonged calcitonin therapy
ay have a favourable effect on the course of the
ne changes.

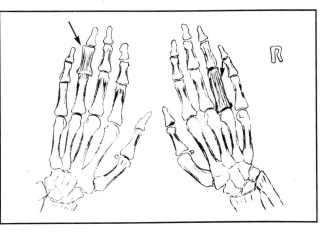

10

11

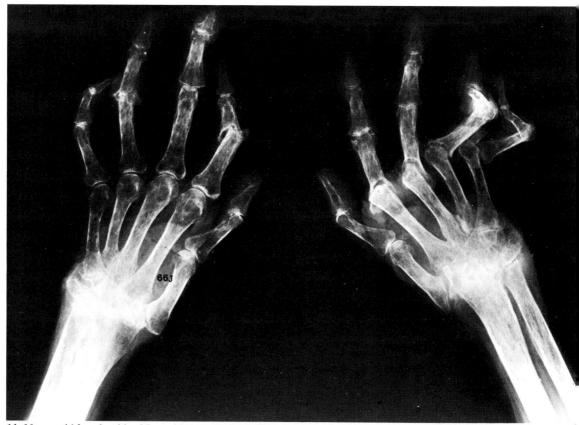

11 66 year-old female with a 25 year history of polyarthritis.

12

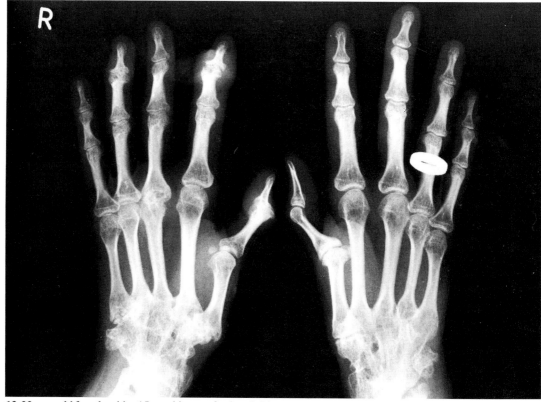

12 22 year-old female with a 15 year history of polyarthritis.

1 Rheumatoid arthritis

·ry progressive form with significant destruc-
n and bone resorption in the region of the
·pus (1), subluxation and ulnar deviation (2),
·ncil cup lesion (3), thin cortex (4).

·s in a small percentage of patients suffering
·m rheumatoid arthritis that the disease pro-
·sses to this degree of infirmity. Prolonged
·rticoid therapy may accelerate progression to
·s stage.

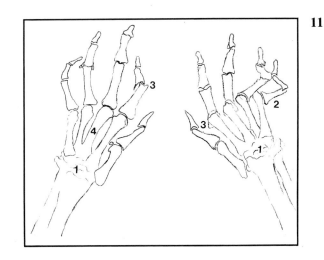

11

2 Non-active juvenile rheumatoid arthritis

·kylosis of the carpus (1), erosion, diminution
·joint space and subluxation (2), sequelae of
·hritis of distal interphalangeal joints with
·perostosis (3).

·kylosis of joints develops faster and more
·ten in juvenile rheumatoid arthritis than in the
·ult form. Care should be taken to maintain the
·flamed joints in a position of function, for
·stance by the application of night splints.

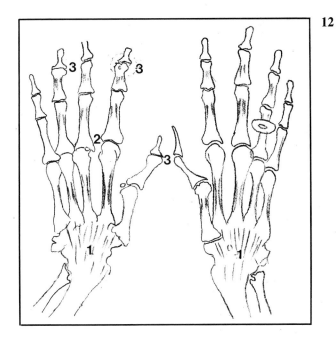

12

13

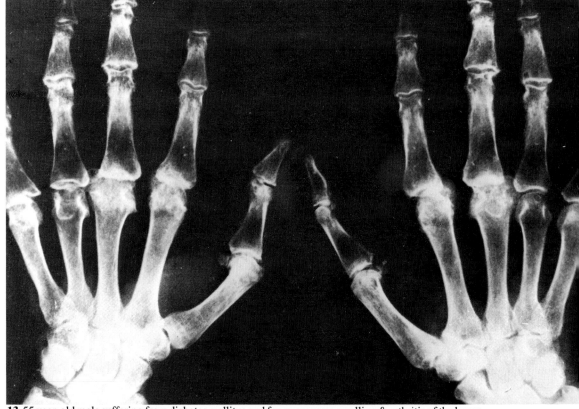

13 55 year-old male suffering from diabetes mellitus and for many years swelling & arthritis of the knees.

14

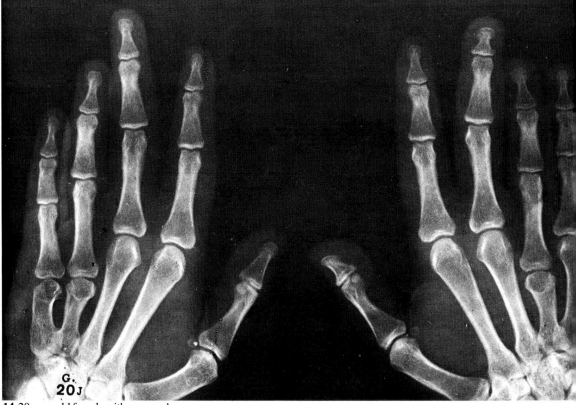

14 20 year-old female with amenorrhoea.

3 Haemochromatosis

symmetrical joint space narrowing (1), hyper-
phy, bone changes at index and middle finger
etacarpophalangeal joints (2), subchondral
stic degeneration (3) and chondrocalcinosis
).

hondrocalcinosis can precede every symptom
haemochromatosis for years. With discovery
a raised serum iron level, timely therapy can be
stituted and prevent damage of the liver, heart
c.

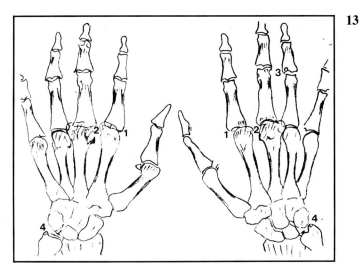

13

4 Turner's syndrome

rachymetacarpia (1), thin cortices and widened
edullary cavities of metacarpals (2).

Turner's syndrome there is an agenesis of the
ary and therefore oestrogen deficiency leading
osteoporosis.
rachymetacarpia also occurs in:
pseudohypoparathyroidism
pseudo-pseudohypoparathyroidism
juvenile rheumatoid arthritis
various rare congenital abnormalities.

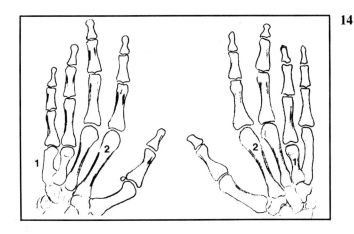

14

15

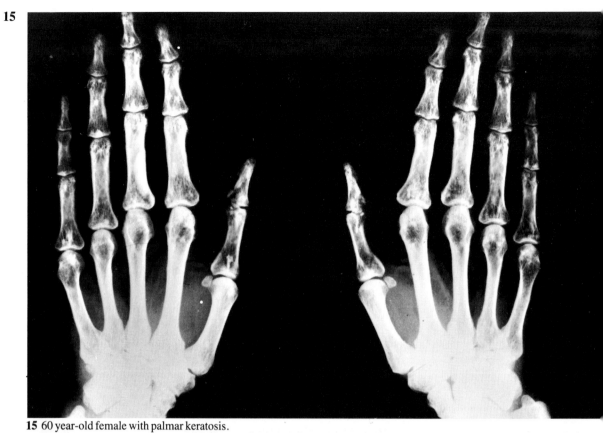

15 60 year-old female with palmar keratosis.

16

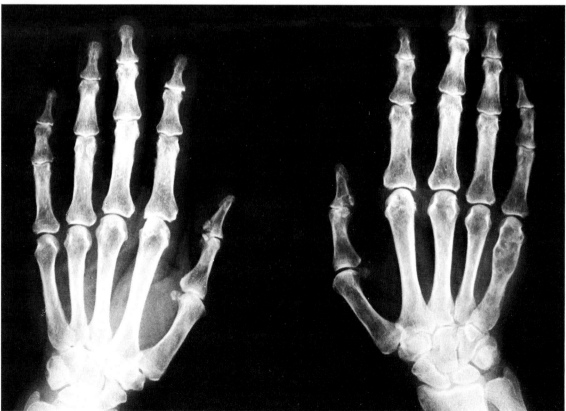

16 63 year-old male with a swelling on the medial border of his right hand.

5 Osteopoikilosis

[M]ultiple foci of sclerotic bone.

[D]ominant autosomal hereditary bone dystrophy [ch]aracterised by multiple foci of dense bone [so]metimes associated with lenticular dermatofib[ro]sis or palmoplantar keratosis. The condition is [as]ymptomatic.

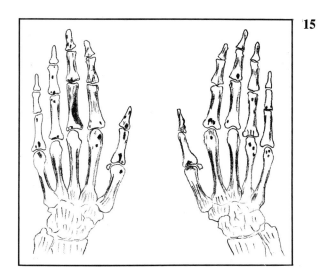
15

6 Enchondroma

[Po]lycystic rarefaction in the diaphysis of the fifth [me]tacarpal with thinning of the cortex and expan[si]on of the medullary cavity (arrow).

[En]chondroma is the commonest benign bone [tu]mour of the hand derived from cartilage rests. [Th]e occurrence of multiple enchondromata, [ch]ondromatosis (usually unilateral) is called [Ol]lier's disease.
  Maffucci's syndrome enchondromata are [as]sociated with haemangiomata of the soft tis[su]es.

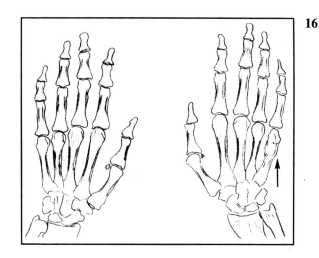
16

17

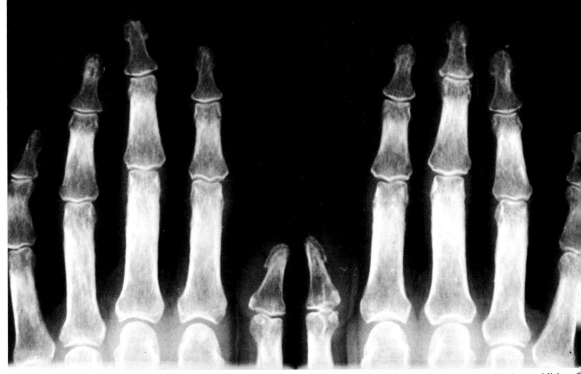

17 55 year-old female with diffuse joint pains without swelling and a long history of Raynaud's syndrome. She has, additionally a pointed nose and telangiectasia of the lips and cheeks.

18

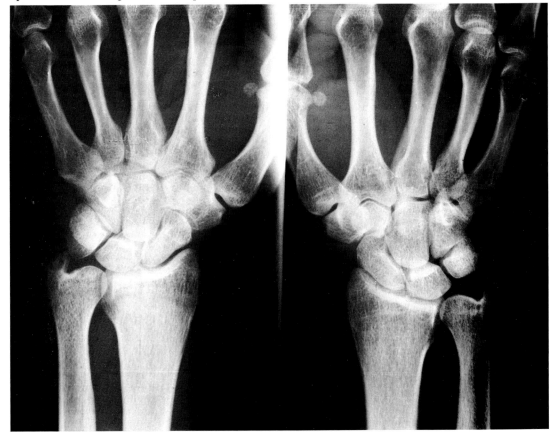

18 35 year-old female with synovial swelling of wrists accompanied by stiffness for an hour each morning.

7 C.R.S.T. syndrome

croosteolysis (1), calcinosis cutis (2).

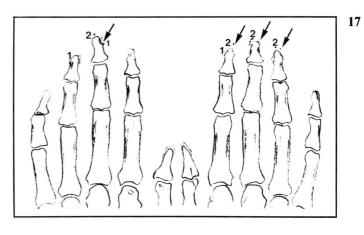

17

ndrome characterised by **C**alcinosis cutis, aynaud's phenomenon, **S**ystemic sclerosis and elangiectasia, hence the name C.R.S.T. synome: a form of systemic sclerosis with a benign urse due to fewer visceral abnormalities than in e classical scleroderma. This syndrome is also own as the Thibièrge-Weissenbach syndrome.

8 Rheumatoid arthritis

rosion of the left styloid process (1), moderate rrowing of the left radiocarpal joint space (2).

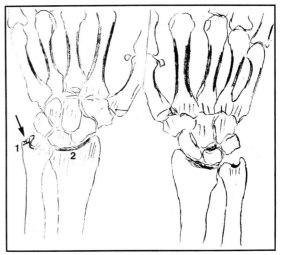

18

rheumatoid arthritis the only sign may be osion of the ulnar styloid or a diastasis of the dioulnar joint. Other clinical signs such as niform synovial swelling, morning stiffness, inful hyperextension or flexion of the joints, bcutaneous nodules and a positive rheumatoid thritis factor in the serum then contribute to the agnosis. No one of these findings on its own is fficient for definite diagnosis.

19

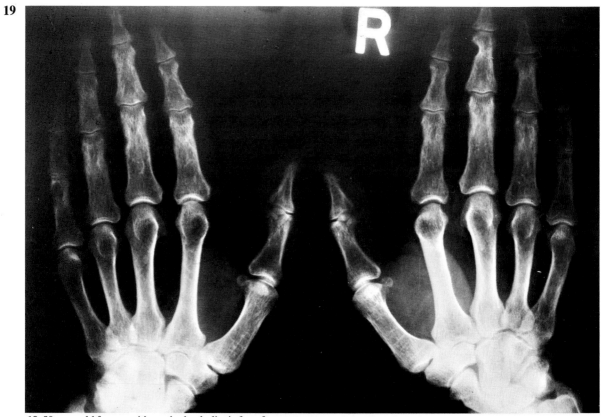

19 50 year-old farmer with marked polydipsia for a few years.

20

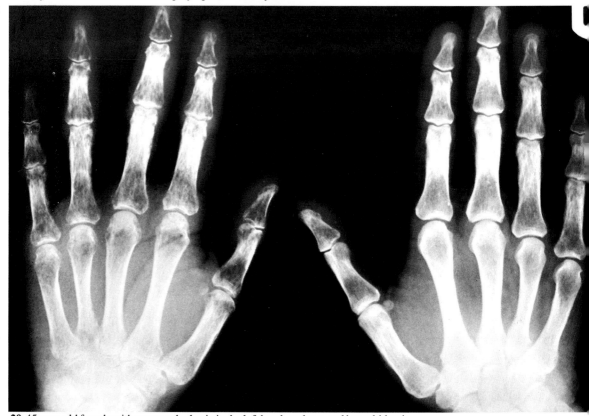

20 45 year-old female with very marked pain in the left hand, oedema and hyperhidrosis.

9 Primary hyperparathyroidism

riosteal bone resorption (1), brown tumour (2),
zy appearance of bone trabeculae (3).

e polydipsia is due to the hypercalcaemia.
ere was also a low blood phosphorus. Asso-
ated kidney stones often occur. Usually the
percalcaemia is asymptomatic and a chance
scovery at examination for some other com-
aint. The disease occurs twice as frequently in
males as in males, especially after the climac-
ric.
e haziness of the bone is due to insufficient
ntrast between the imperfectly calcified bone
d the soft tissues.

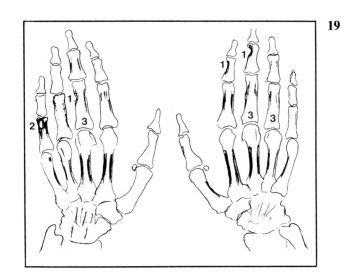

19

0 Algoneurodystrophy

ffuse osteoporosis and patchy bone structure of
e left hand.

llowing trauma which may be insignificant, a
vere pain syndrome ensues with marked
steoporosis, vasomotor disturbances and
ophic signs of the soft tissues.
e syndrome has also been called sympathetic
godystrophy. Re-education is the most impor-
nt form of treatment.

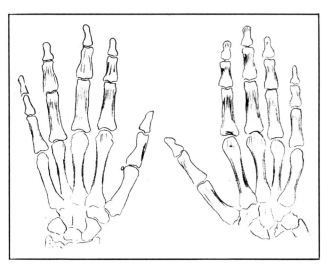

20

21

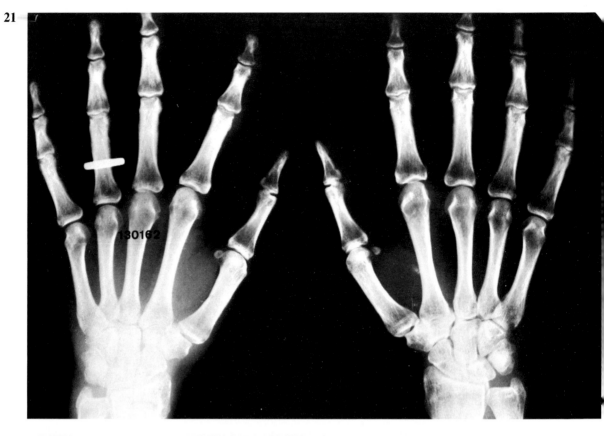

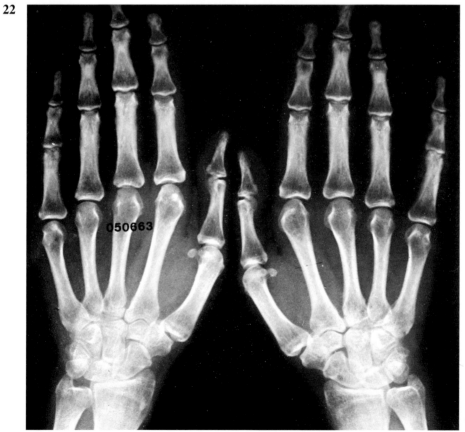

◄**21** 30 year-old female wi
symmetrical joint swellings
of hands, feet and knees
for two years.

◄**22** 18 months later.

21 Rheumatoid arthritis: Stage II

Arthritis of left middle finger metacarpopha-langeal joint with periarticular osteoporosis (1), joint space narrowing (2), and marginal erosions (3). Dense appearance of the carpus due to synovial thickening (4).

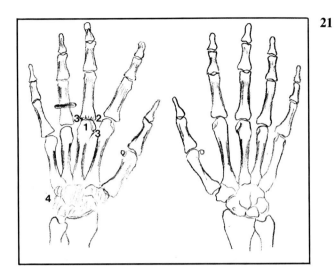

21

22 Rheumatoid arthritis: Stage II

Arthritis of left middle finger metacarpopha-langeal joint (1), early joint space narrowing of right and left radiocarpal joints (2), and second and third right metacarpophalangeal joints (3), cystic translucency right carpus (4).

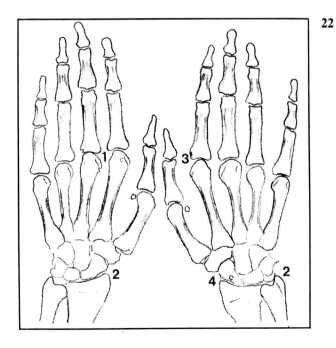

22

23

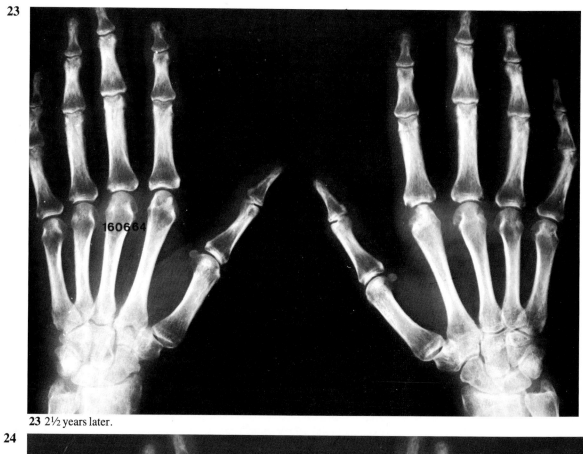

23 2½ years later.

24

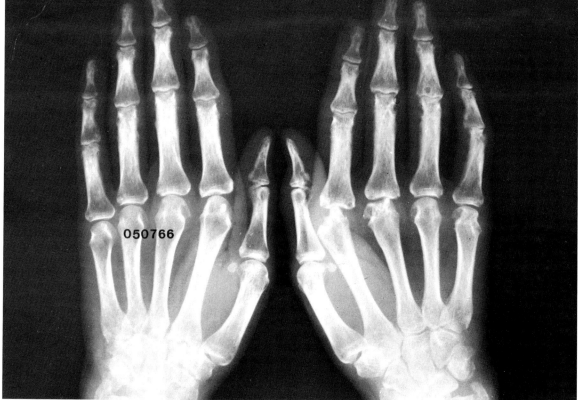

24 4½ years later.

3 Rheumatoid arthritis: Stage III

osive arthritis of the left middle finger metacar-
phalangeal joint, right index and middle finger
etacarpophalangeal joints and right proximal
terphalangeal joint (1), radiocarpal and inter-
rpal joint space narrowing, right as well as left
), irregular bone structure of the ulnar styloid (3).

23

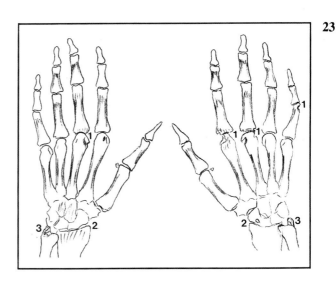

4 Rheumatoid arthritis: Stage IV

osive destruction of the carpal joints on the left
), lower end of radius (2), styloid process of the
na (3), carpometacarpal joints (4), narrowing of
diocarpal joint space (5), erosive arthritis left
iddle finger and right index and middle finger
etacarpophalangeal joints (6), early erosions of
ads of right ring and little finger metacarpals
), arthritis proximal interphalangeal joints of
ght middle, ring and little fingers (8).

24

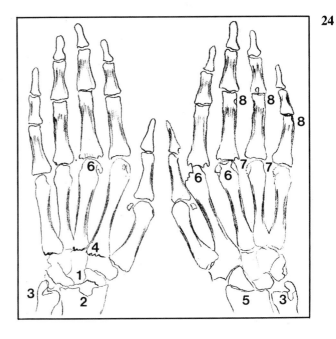

25

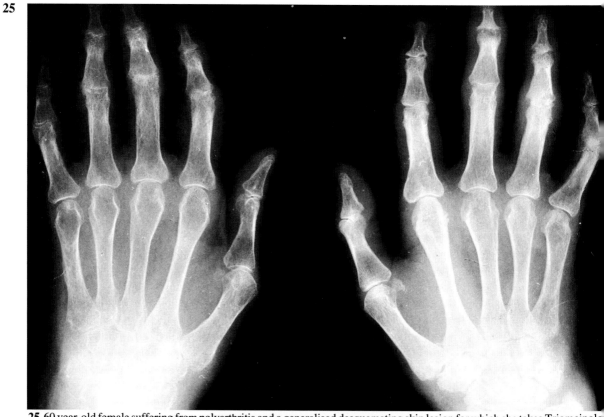

25 60 year-old female suffering from polyarthritis and a generalised desquamating skin lesion for which she takes Triamcinolo

26

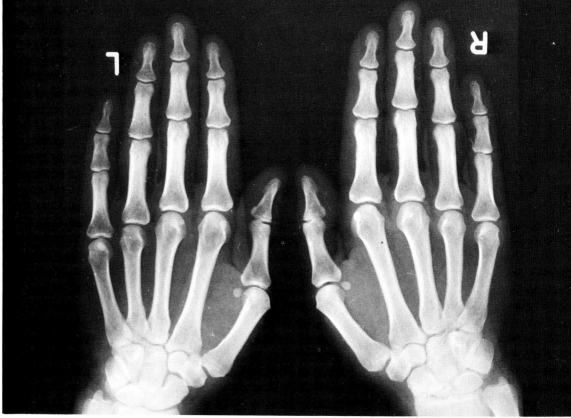

26 30 year-old female secretary complaining of pain in the right wrist.

25 Psoriatic arthritis

Involvement of distal interphalangeal (1), proximal interphalangeal (2), metacarpophalangeal joints (3), ankylosis of left wrist (4).

The involvement of the distal interphalangeal joints is typical of psoriatic arthritis. As a rule the nails are then also affected. The skin lesions may be discrete. In rare cases psoriatic arthritis may lead to artritis mutilans. The polyarthritis of psoriasis is often difficult to distinguish from rheumatoid polyarthritis.
The rheumatoid arthritis factor is absent in psoriatic arthritis.

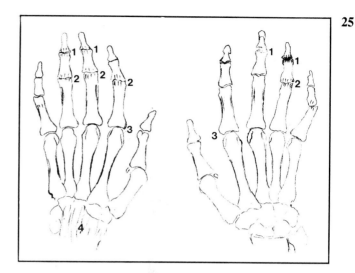

25

26 Aseptic necrosis of the scaphoid

Irregular structure of the right scaphoid (arrow) with secondary narrowing of the radiocarpal joint space.

Monoarticular pain of the mechanical type should always remind one of the sequelae of trauma with anatomical changes. A careful comparison with the bone structure of the unaffected hand brings the lesion to light.

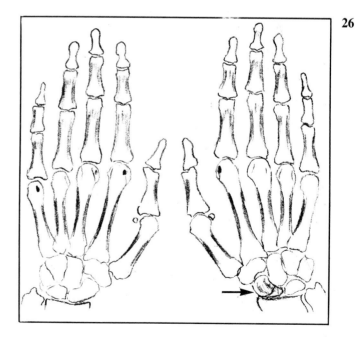

26

27

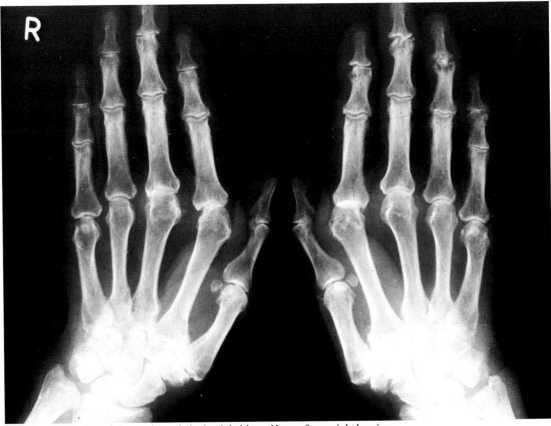

27 70 year-old lady with increasing pain in the right hip and knee after weight bearing.

28

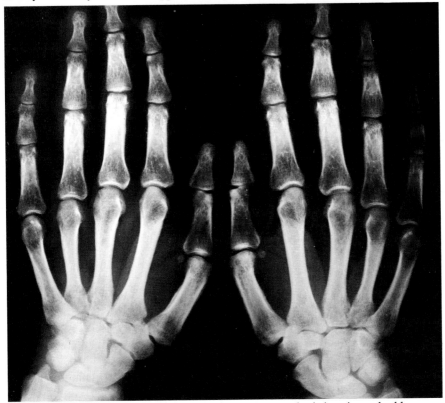

28 43 year-old male with drumstick fingers and severe nocturnal pain in wrists and ankles.

7 Polyarthrosis

regular narrowing of joint cavities, osteophyto-s, subchondral sclerosis and cystic translucen-es (1), subluxation of the root of the thumb (rhizarthrosis) (2).

Polyarthrosis of the small joints of the hand affects particularly the distal, proximal and meta-carpal joints. The wrist joints are usually spared. Polyarthrosis indicates a hereditary arthropathic diathesis also involving other joints: hips, knees, feet and vertebral column.

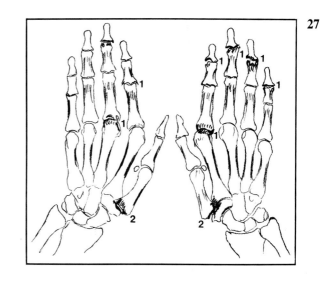

27

8 Hypertrophic pulmonary osteoarthropathy, Pierre-Marie-Bamberger's disease

Periosteal reaction in right and left thumb meta-carpal (arrows).

Intrathoracic tumours, especially bronchogenic carcinoma, give rise to this abnormality. The clinical picture may be confused with rheumatoid arthritis. The drumstick fingers however point to intrathoracic pathology. The complaint dis-appears after extirpation of the tumour.

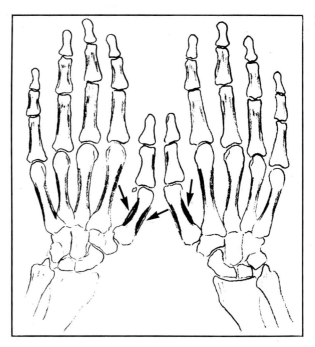

28

29

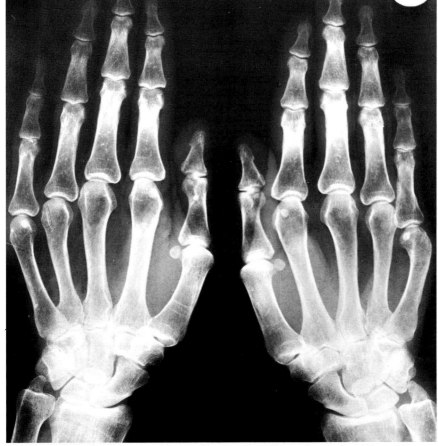

29 50 year-old male with a recent history of a traumatic collapse of a vertebra, bilateral fractured neck of femur and fractured clavicle.

30

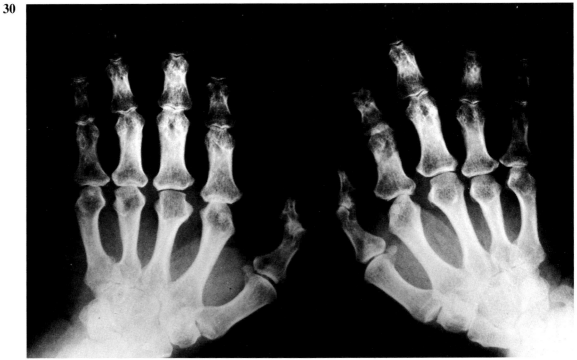

30 40 year-old remarkably short female.

29 Idiopathic osteoporosis

Thin cortex and widened medullary cavities of the metacarpals (1), growth arrest lines (2), healed fracture of right fifth metacarpal (3).

Osteoporosis is differentiated radiologically from osteomalacia by the sharply outlined bone structure.

In osteomalacia the bone structure is vague owing to the weak calcification of the bone matrix. There are clear biochemical differences between osteoporosis and osteomalacia. In osteoporosis the parameters of bone metabolism are normal, but they are altered in the case of osteomalacia; for instance low blood calcium and phosphate as well as increased alkaline phosphatase activity.

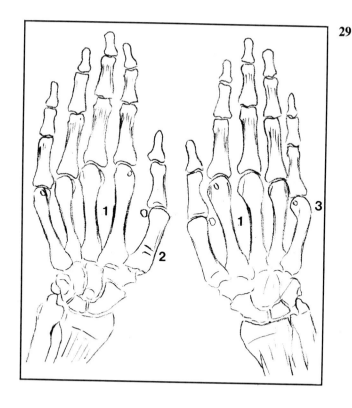

30 Achondroplasia

Short, thick metacarpals and phalanges, with widened ends. Metacarpal heads are pointed. Deformity of the ulna.

Achondroplasia is an autosomal dominant genetic disorder with dwarfism due to incomplete proliferation of growth cartilage. The limbs are short, the trunk length nearly normal. Spinal cord compression with paraplegia often occurs as well as secondary arthropathy of the hips.

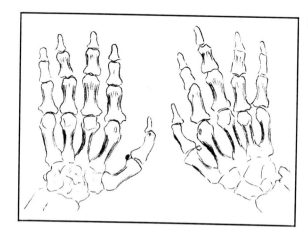

31

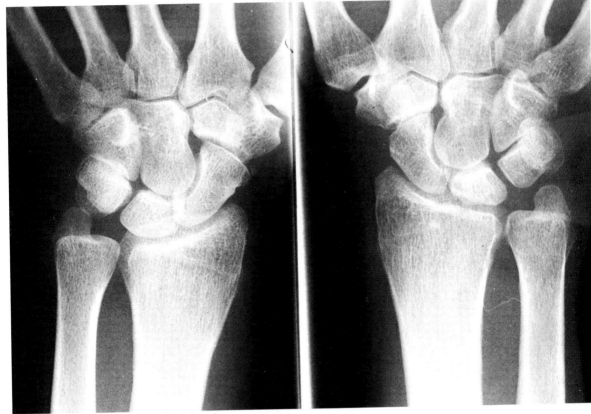

31 47 year-old male with pain in the right wrist.

32

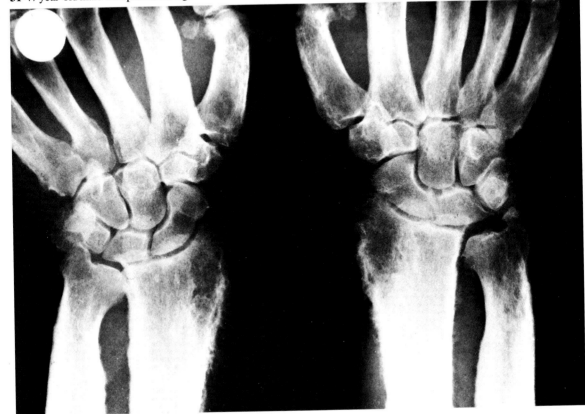

32 55 year-old male with very clumsy limbs.

31 Aseptic necrosis of the lunate

Flattening and uneven opacity of the lunate (arrow).

This condition is also called Kienböck's osteochondritis or osteochondrosis. It is usually the result of trauma but often there is no history of injury.

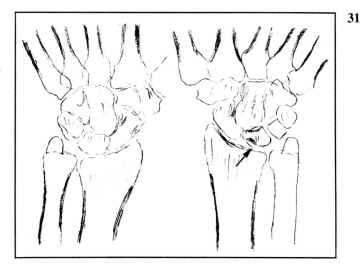

31

32 Pachydermoperiostosis

Marked periostosis of radius and ulna. Wide, irregular metacarpals.

Pachydermoperiostosis is a hereditary familial condition characterised by a thick skin and manifest periostosis. The radiological picture has to be distinguished from the periostosis occurring with intrathoracic tumours.

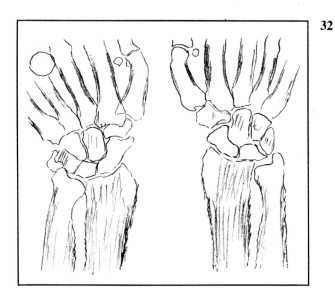

32

33

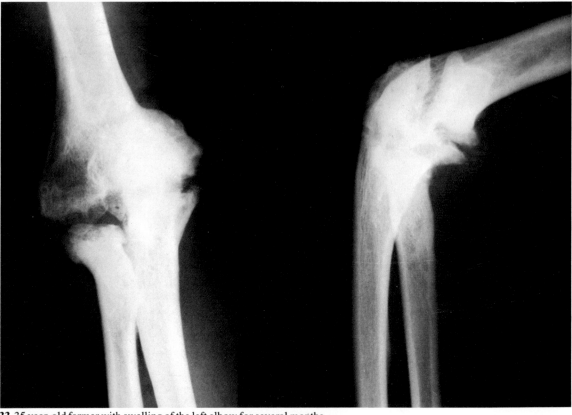

33 35 year-old farmer with swelling of the left elbow for several months.

34

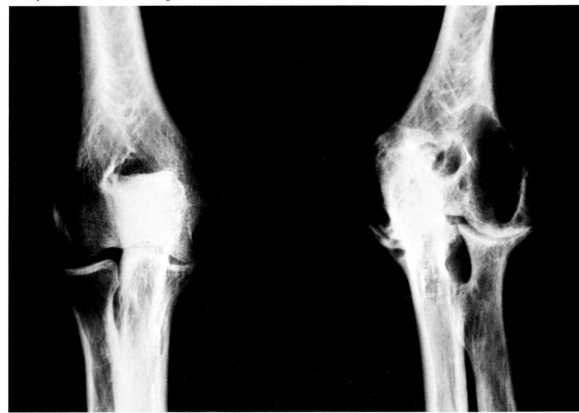

34 40 year-old male with polyarthritis for 7 years. Paralysis of the right arm for 20 years due to traumatic nerve injury.

3 Tuberculous arthritis

arked joint destruction with margin erosions.

monoarthritis persisting for several months
ould always arouse suspicion of tuberculous
novitis. Often a synovial biopsy is necessary to
onfirm the diagnosis.

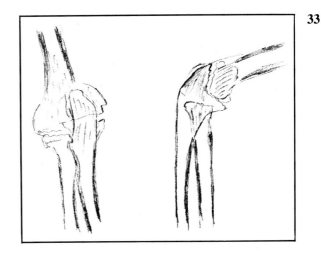

33

4 Rheumatoid arthritis

rave destruction of the left elbow (1), with
condary osteophytosis (2) and a giant cyst (3).

he right elbow shows no radiological lesion.
he signs of rheumatoid arthritis are less obvious
 paralysed limbs, emphasising the importance
f mechanical influences on the destructive
rocess.

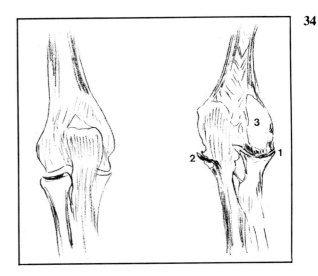

34

35

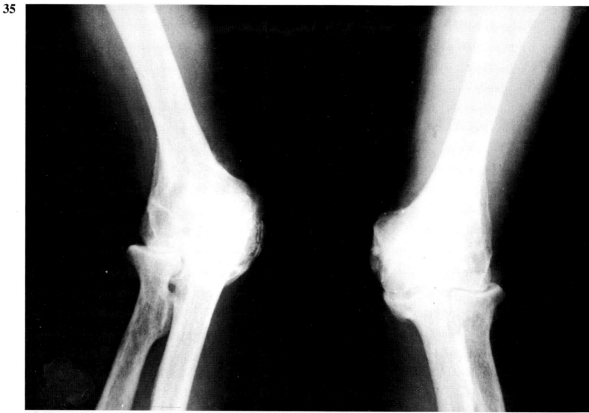

35 53 year-old dairy farmer with pain in the elbows.

36

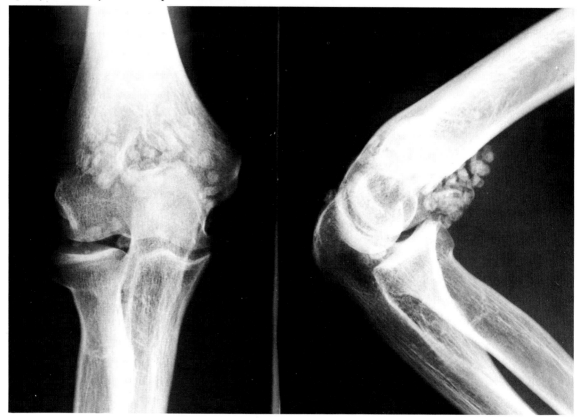

36 23 year-old male complaining of recurrent locking of the elbow.

35 Secondary arthropathy

Capsular calcification (1), osteophytosis (2), sclerotic reaction and limitation of extension.

Arthropathy of the elbow is almost always the result of trauma or microtrauma as often occurs in pneumatic drill workers.

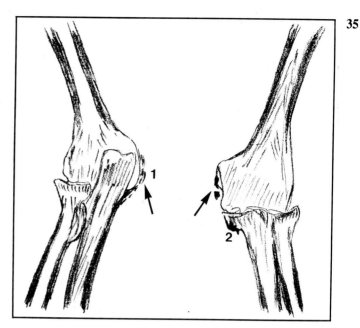

36 Synovial osteochondromatosis

Multiple free intrasynovial osteocartilaginous bodies.

Synovial osteochondromatosis is a painless, chronic monoarticular condition giving rise to locking of the joint and sometimes arthropathy. The intra-articular bodies are originally cartilaginous and therefore radiotranslucent. They calcify and tend to increase in size. They are often the result of trauma.

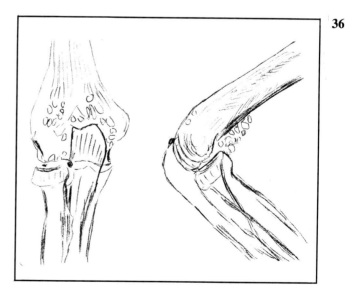

37

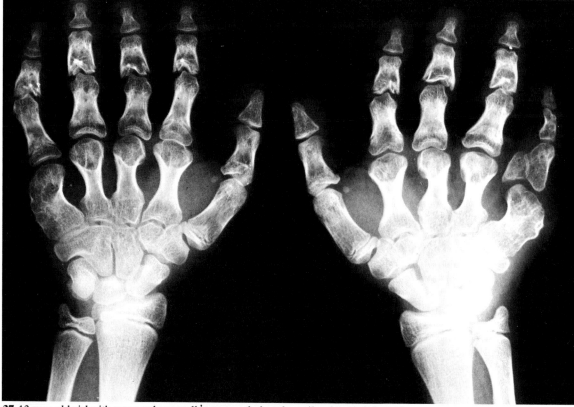

37 13 year-old girl with genua valga, small stature, polydactyly, nail and tooth deformities.

38

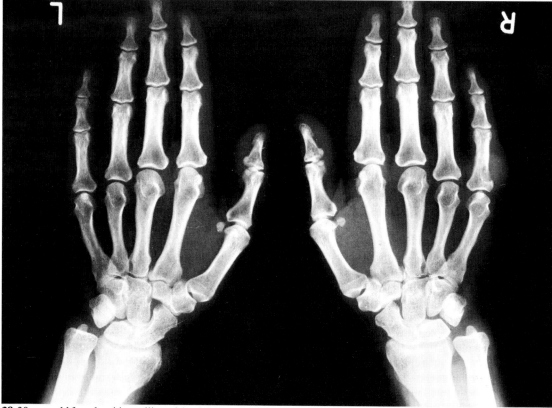

38 30 year-old female with swelling of the right little finger.

37 Chondroectodermal dysplasia, Ellis-Van Crefeld disease

Shortening of the metacarpal and phalangeal shafts, with conical shape; remains of earlier polydactyly (operated) near the fifth metacarpal.

Rare recessive autosomal condition characterised by: dwarfism due to shortness of the long bones distal to knee and elbow, micromelia, polydactyly, hypoplasia of teeth and nails. Congenital heart disease occurs in 60 per cent of cases.

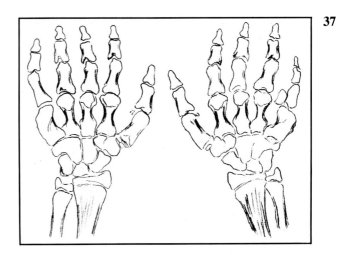

37

38 Villonodular synovitis

Epiphyseal geode and soft tissue swelling of the proximal phalanx of the little finger (arrow).

Villonodular synovitis is almost always monoarticular and involves particularly the knee, ankle, shoulder and rarely the hip. Histologically, the synovitis is characterised by fibroblastic tissue with fat-laden histiocytes, haemosiderin and giant cells.

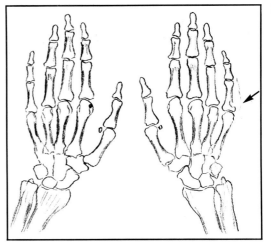

38

39

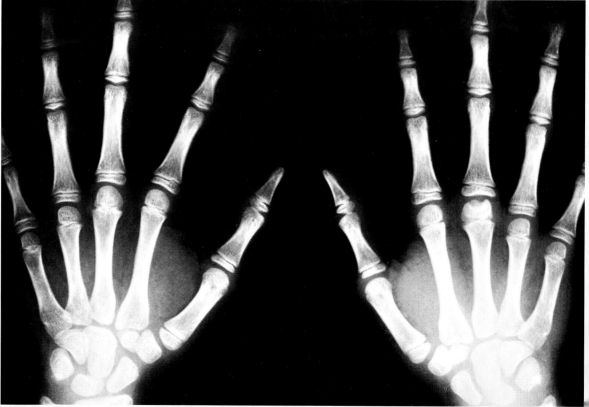

39 12 year-old boy with swelling of the dorsum of his right hand.

40

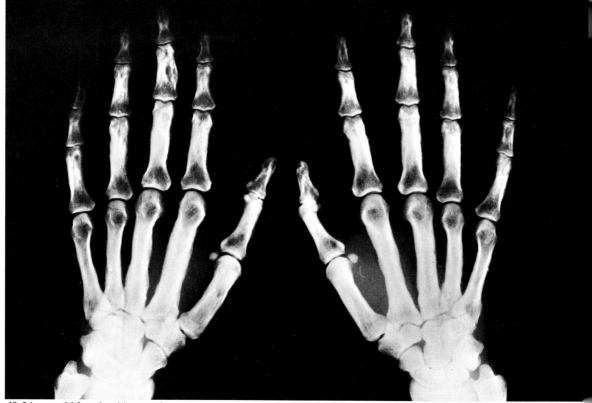

40 24 year-old female with mental retardation.

39 Osteochondrosis of the head of the right middle finger metacarpal

Halfmoon shaped lacunae with sclerosis of the margins (arrow).

Growth abnormality resulting in aseptic necrosis. Occurs infrequently in the hands. May later lead to secondary arthropathy.

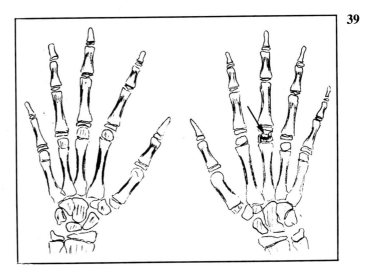

39

40 Tuberous sclerosis

Periosteal thickening of the metacarpals with sclerosis, irregular bone structure of the middle phalanx of the left middle finger with lacunar areas and sclerosis.

Tuberous sclerosis is a rare congenital mesoneurectodermal abnormality with bony sclerosis, skin lesions, brain tumours and many other abnormalities.

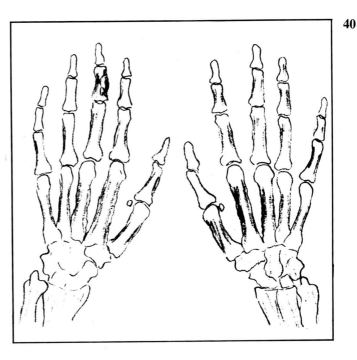

40

2: The vertebral column

The vertebral column occupies a unique place in the skeleton. Its role in the erect position is indispensable; it protects and channels much of the nervous system and by virtue of its principally cancellous composition is intimately involved in metabolic and haemopoietic processes. In appraising radiographs of this region it is as well to be aware of all these functions.

Pain in the vertebral column and alteration in the bony structure can be ascribed to many different causes. The vertebral column is not only the seat of numerous benign degenerative processes but often constitutes the primary site of haemopoietic disease or metastasis. Anatomical curvatures as well as the super-imposition of other organs render the evaluation of a radiograph of the vertebral column less straightforward. The presence of anatomical curvatures calls for specific radiographs taken from suitably adjusted angles. Examination of skeletal structures on radiographs taken for the stomach or kidneys is dangerous because various shadows, incorrectly interpreted as pathological, may occur on them.

41

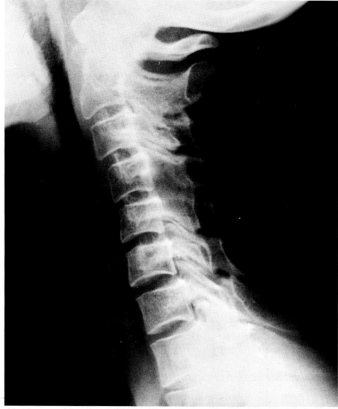

41 19 year-old patient with swelling of the wrist for 5 years.

42

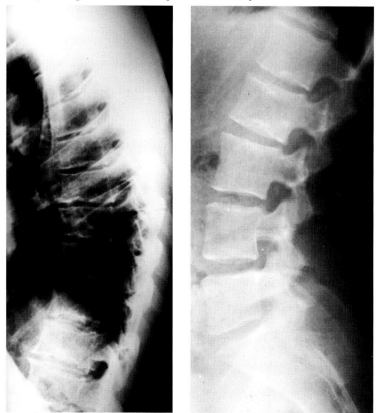

42 Dressmaker, aged 28, experiencing pain in the interscapular region in the evening.

41 Juvenile rheumatoid arthritis

Rigid cervical spine with ankylosis of the C4-C5 apophyseal articulation and periarticular osteoporosis.

In 30 per cent of cases of juvenile rheumatoid arthritis the disease remains oligo- or monoarticular. Involvement of the vertebral column is usually confined to the cervical apophyseal joints. This lesion is often asymptomatic. Polyarthritis in children accompanied by fever, especially in the evening and with systemic involvement, is called Still-Chauffard disease.

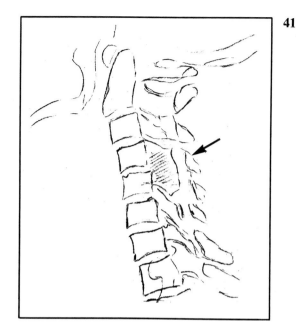

41

42 Scheuermann's disease

Moderate thoracic kyphosis, uneven plane surfaces of vertebral bodies (1), wedge shaped bodies of the middle thoracic vertebrae (2), anterior osteophytosis (3), Schmorl's nodules (4).

Scheuermann's disease, often called juvenile vertebral epiphysitis, is a condition of unknown origin, characterised by irregular development of thoracic and upper lumbar vertebrae. There is irregular ossification of the epiphyseal ring of the vertebral body. The condition is usually painless and associated with curvature of the spine which develops gradually.

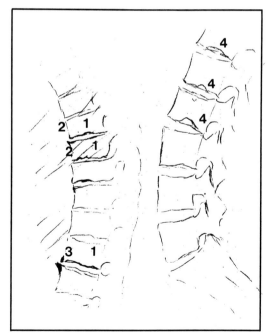

42

43

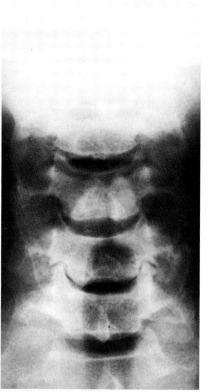
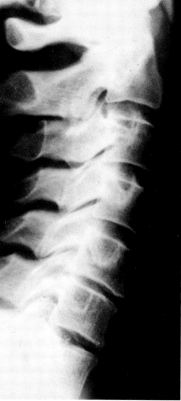
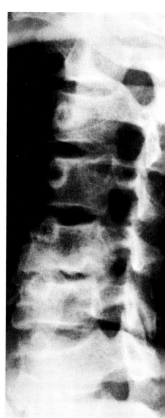

43 45 year-old cobbler complaining of pain in his right arm and paraesthesia of the right hand.

44

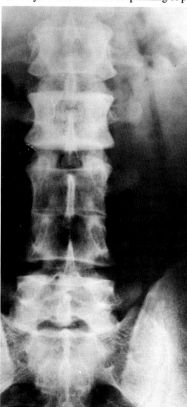
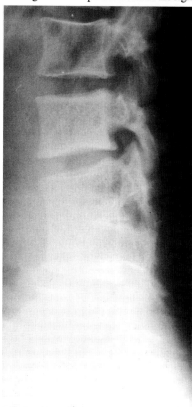

44 Architect of 39 years. Acute lumbago.

43 Cervical arthropathy

ttenuated intervertebral disc C5-C6 (1) with
ncal arthropathy (2) and narrowing of the inter-
ertebral foramen (3).

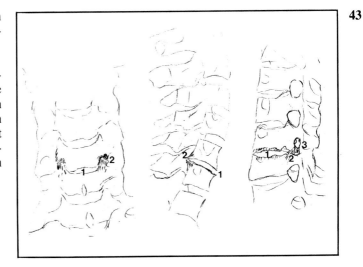

43

ervical arthropathy frequently appears at a re-
tively early age. The painful manifestations are
ery sporadic and do not correlate absolutely with
ne radiological deformities. A pain originating in
ne shoulder region and radiating to the neck must
ot be confused with a cervical arthropathy, de-
nite the presence of radiological abnormalities in
ne cervical spine.

44 Haemangioma – congenital vertebral fusion

Haemangioma of L2 vertebra, coarse trabecular
tructure with vertical striation (1), fusion of the
bodies of L3 and L4 vertebrae with disc hypopla-
ia (2).

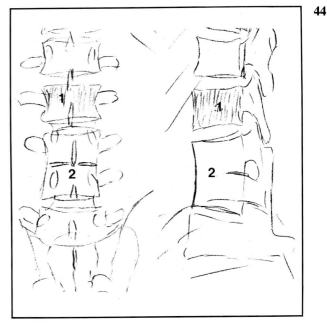

44

A haemangioma often appears in the vertebral
column and is usually asymptomatic. Very rarely
vertebral collapse may occur. The affected ver-
ebra is not expanded and can thus be differentiated from Paget's disease. The vertical
striation distinguishes a haemangioma from a
solitary vertebral metastasis.

Congenital fusion results from incomplete
separation of two vertebrae with, as a result, a
hypoplastic disc and anterior angulation. In the
adult such a deformity is difficult to distinguish
from the outcome of a spondylodiscitis. The
fusion alters the normal distribution of force to the
intervertebral discs, resulting in overloading and
degeneration of the adjacent discs above or
below.

45

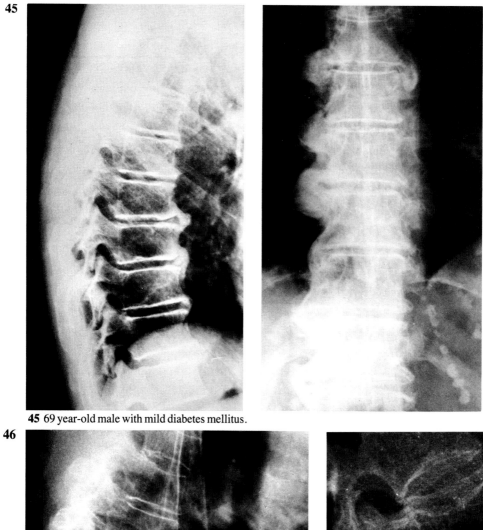

45 69 year-old male with mild diabetes mellitus.

46

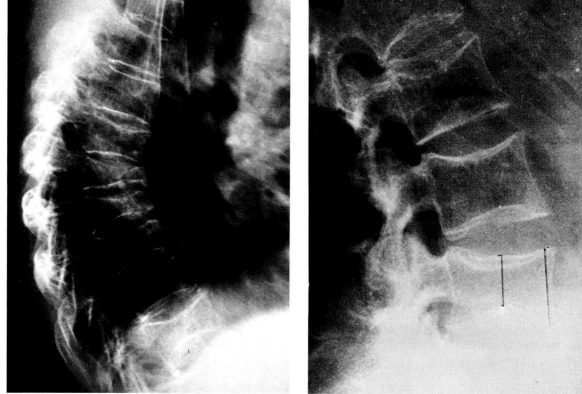

46 65 year-old female with a few years history of pain in the back radiating in girdle pattern to the chest and groins; pain on turning over in bed.

5 Hyperostosis vertebralis

[bo]ny intervertebral bridges along the right side of [th]e thoracic spine.

[Hy]perostosis vertebralis is a specific form of [sp]ondylosis occurring in the elderly, particularly [ma]les. Forestier described this deformity as 'an[ky]losing vertebral hyperostosis of the aged'.

[Th]e radiological picture resembles that found in [an]kylosing spondylitis with overgrown, some[ti]mes enormous, calcifications of the lateral and [an]terior intervertebral ligaments without in[vo]lvement of the sacroiliac joints. The vertebral [col]umn is rigid but practically always painless. A [mi]ld diabetes mellitus is often associated.

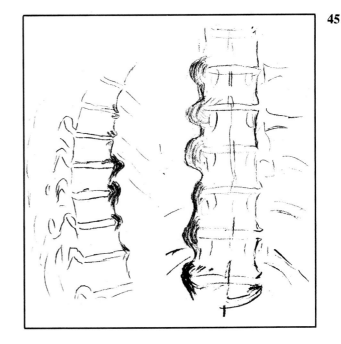

45

6 Primary axial osteoporosis

[W]edge shaped flattening of the vertebral bodies [in] the mid-thoracic region (1), diabolo vertebrae [in] lumbar region (2), biconcavity index (3): h/H [ex]pressed in % = 65% (normally more than [80]%).

[Pr]imary axial osteoporosis occurs particularly in [po]stclimacteric women. It rarely occurs in young [pa]tients and is then called idiopathic axial [os]teoporosis. Secondary osteoporosis is found [af]ter corticosteroid and heparin administration, [im]mobilisation, gastrectomy, castration, hyper[pa]rathyroidism, hyperthyroidism and long[sta]nding arthritis. With advancing age, after 40, [th]ere is physiological diminution of bone mass, [m]ore obvious in women than in men. Loss of bone [m]ass in women after 40 is about 1 per cent per [ye]ar.

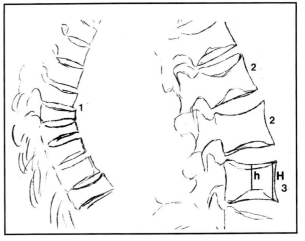

46

47

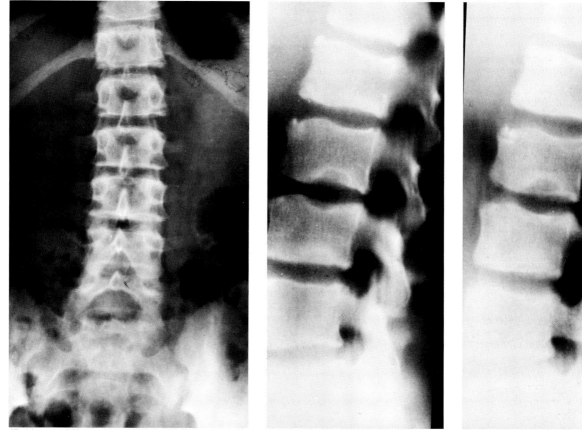

47 14 year-old boy with a 6 month history of pain and stiffness of the back, particularly in the morning. Despite a negative Manto he was treated with tuberculostatic agents.

48

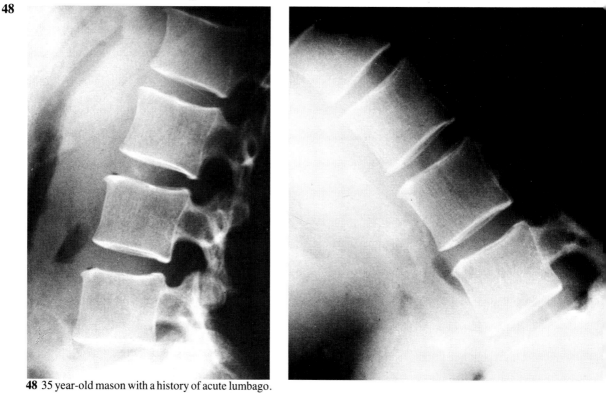

48 35 year-old mason with a history of acute lumbago.

47 Nonspecific spondylodiscitis

Uniform narrowing of L2-L3 disc (1), central osteolysis of adjacent vertebral bodies (2) particularly evident on tomography, hazy and broadened sacroiliac joint space (3).

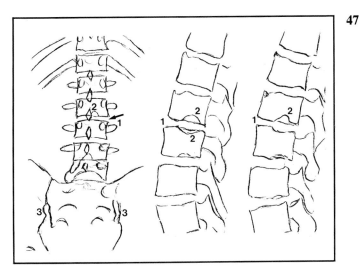

A spondylodiscitis heralding the onset of ankylosing spondylitis (Bechterew's disease) is difficult to distinguish radiologically from tuberculous spondylodiscitis. In young patients, the assessment of the sacroiliac joint is similarly difficult. In children the sacroiliac joint cavity is normally wide and not sharply demarcated.

48 Disc degeneration – spondylosis

Vacuum phenomenon (1), slight narrowing of discs L2-L3 and L3-L4 (2) with early osteophytosis of the margins (3).

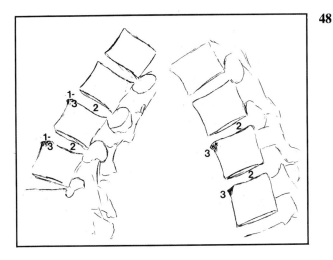

The vacuum phenomenon is a translucent area produced by gas aspirated from interstitial fluid by negative pressure brought about in a space abnormally opened by hyperextension.

This phenomenon appears only in areas of disc degeneration. The vacuum phenomenon disappears with flexion. This sign can be used as a test for disc disease. Narrowing of the disc space may be the only sign of disc disease. Normally the disc spaces in the lumbar region increase in height from L1 to L5. Disc space L5-S1 is normally narrower than that of L4-L5.

49

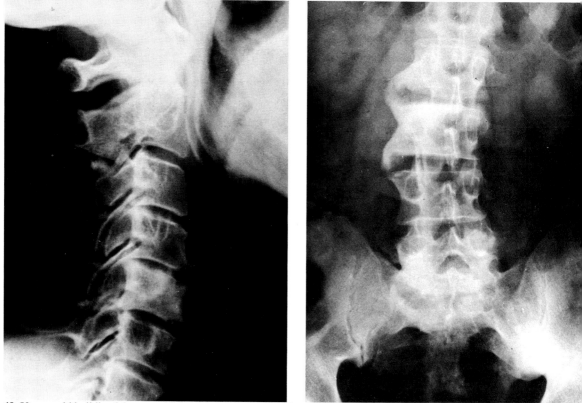

49 50 year-old building labourer with hyperkeratosis of the palms and soles; periods of very bad backache. History of iritis and urethral dilatations.

50

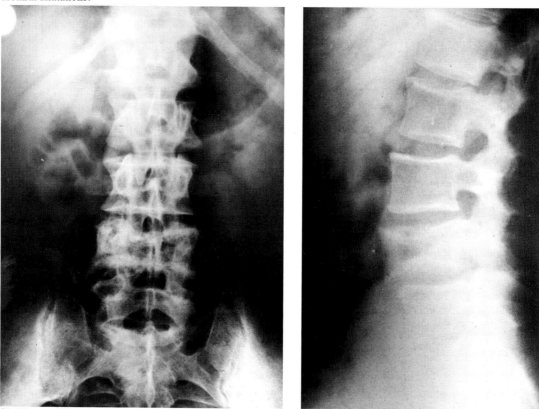

50 55 year-old female with vague backache especially at night, radiating to both lower limbs.

49 Pelvispondylitis in a case of Reiter's syndrome

Osteitis of vertebral body C5 (1), asymmetrical osteitis of L2-L3 giving the appearance of a cow's horns (2), arthritis of the lower third of the right sacroiliac joint (3).

Reiter's syndrome, also called Fiessinger-Leroy syndrome in the French literature, is characterised by the triad urethritis, arthritis and conjunctivitis. These three maladies frequently appear at different times and may follow an attack of dysentery.

Other equally important signs are circinate balanitis, superficial ulceration of the cheek mucous membrane (aphthosis) and a characteristic dermatitis (keratoderma blennorrhagica). Unlike the peripheral joint lesions, the spondylitis of Reiter's syndrome may remain active for years.

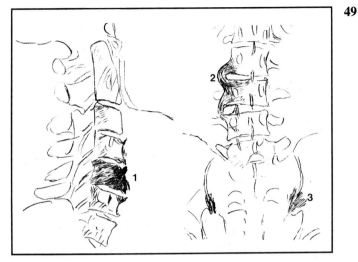

49

50 Paget's disease

Picture frame vertebra L4, widening in comparison with neighbouring vertebrae, reduction in height and asymmetry; abnormal trabecular pattern producing an image resembling a picture frame.

In Paget's disease (osteitis deformans) the vertebral lesion is usually asymptomatic. Increased width of a vertebra may exert pressure on the spinal cord or cause radiculopathy. In this disease the bone structure is poor and may therefore lead to fracture or deformity.

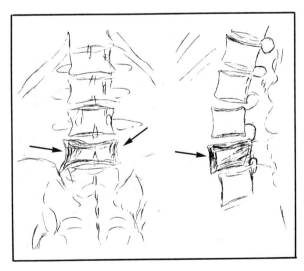

50

51

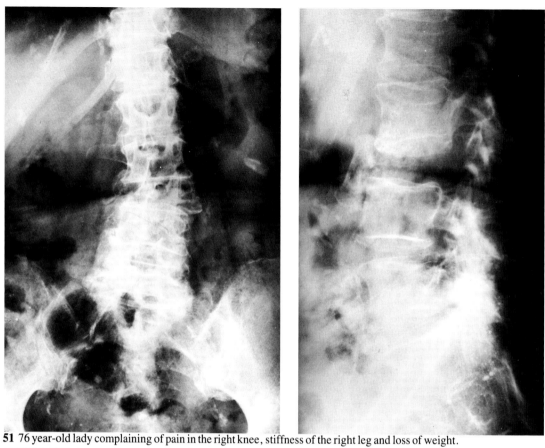

51 76 year-old lady complaining of pain in the right knee, stiffness of the right leg and loss of weight.

52

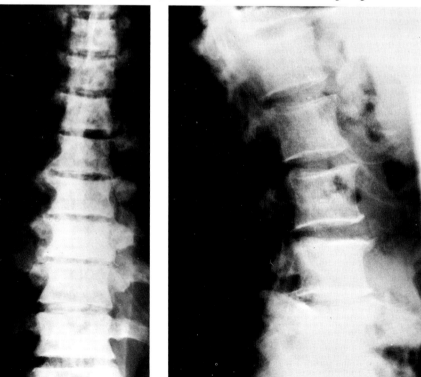

52 73 year-old pensioner employee with day and night lumbosacral pain and poor general condition. At the age of 40 he had a gastrectomy, at 42 a cholecystectomy and at 70, a prostatectomy.

51 Multiple myelomatosis or Kahler's disease

Severe osteolysis of L3 vertebral body and right pedicle L3.

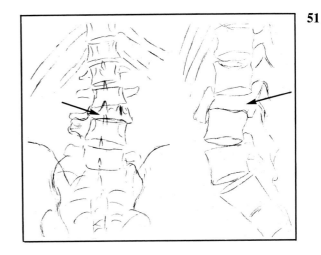

51

The bone lesions of multiple myeloma can present many different forms, either a generalised osteoporosis of the vertebral column, discrete rarefied areas or localised lysis of a vertebra with collapse. Involvement of a pedicle is rare in myelomatosis in contrast with metastasis which selectively affects the pedicle first. There is a grossly raised E.S.R., serum protein electrophoresis shows an increased gamma globulin fraction with monoclonal band, and on sternal puncture one finds massive plasmocytosis. Some cases show hypercalcaemia. Cytostatic treatment of Kahler's disease has improved the five year survival rate considerably.

52 Osteoblastic bone metastases of prostatic carcinoma

Dense shadows (1), unevenly spread over the whole vertebral column with here and there the picture of an ivory vertebra (2), osteophytosis (3).

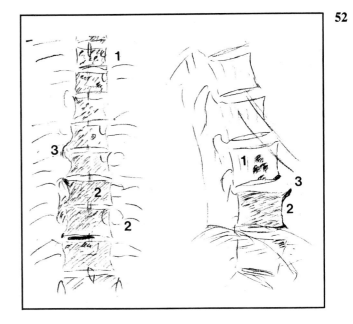

52

Osteoblastic bone secondaries occur mainly with carcinoma of the prostate, breast, lung and stomach. Osteoblastic metastasis of prostatic carcinoma is usually accompanied by a raised serum acid phosphatase. Treatment is still possible at this stage and may produce a prolonged remission.

53

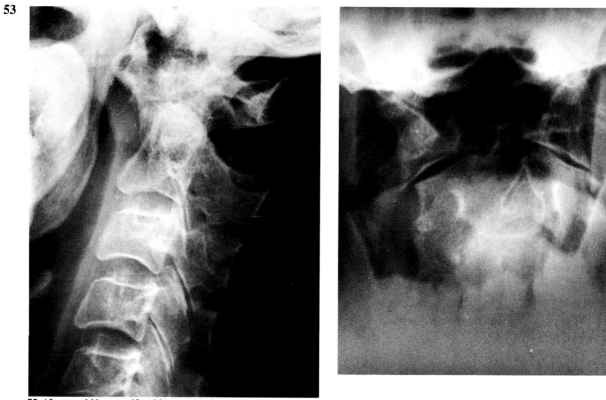

53 45 year-old housewife with severe polyarthritis for 10 years and slightly restricted neck rotation.

54

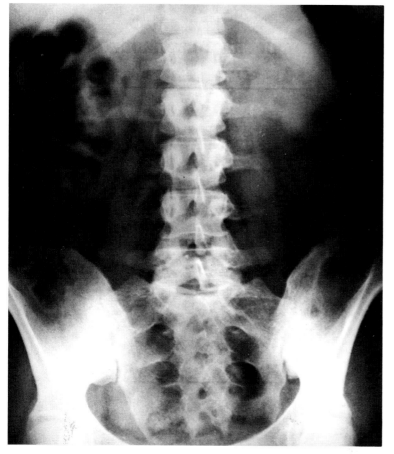

54 30 year-old housewife with low backache for 6 months particularly at night and after rest. She has had a desquamating area of the scalp for a considerable time.

53 Rheumatoid arthritis – atlantoaxial subluxation

Subluxation of C1-C2 (1) in the sagittal plane. The anterior arch of the atlas is displaced forward more than 3mm in relation to the anterior surface of the dens (often only visible on a picture taken in flexion).

On the plate taken through the mouth, one sees erosions on the dens (2), joint space narrowing of the lateral atlantoaxial joint (3) and subluxation in the frontal plane (4).

Atlantoaxial subluxation occurs in 25 per cent of cases with severe rheumatoid arthritis, being usually asymptomatic, with no neurological signs. The space between the atlas and the dens is normally not more than 3mm. Manipulation of the neck in patients with rheumatoid arthritis, particularly under anaesthesia, can be fatal.

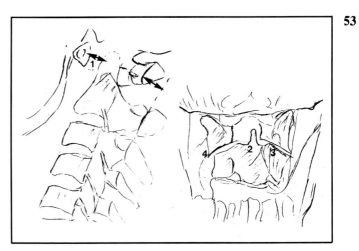

54 Psoriatic spondylitis

Parasyndesmophyte on the right of L2-L3 (1), irregular margins and slight sclerosis of the sacroiliac joints (2).

In psoriasis, spondylitis may occur as well as peripheral arthritis, especially in patients who possess the human leucocyte antigen (HLA) B27.

Radiologically one observes, besides signs of sacroiliitis, a parasyndesmophyte, that is, a detached ligamentous calcification. Similar parasyndesmophytes are also seen in Reiter's syndrome. Moreover the skin lesion of Reiter's syndrome, keratoderma blennorrhagica, is often not easily distinguishable from psoriasis pustulosa.

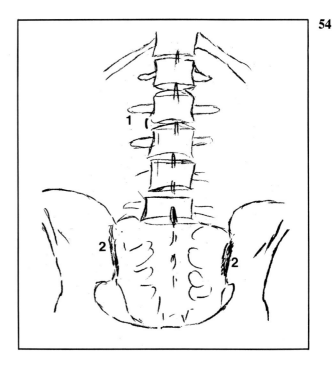

55

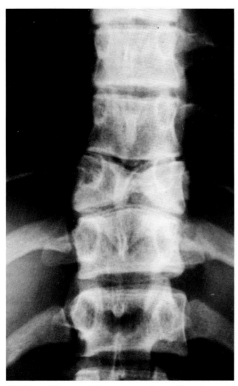

55 In an 18 year-old garage worker with epigastric pain, an abnormality of the spine is discovered during radiographic examination of the stomach.

56

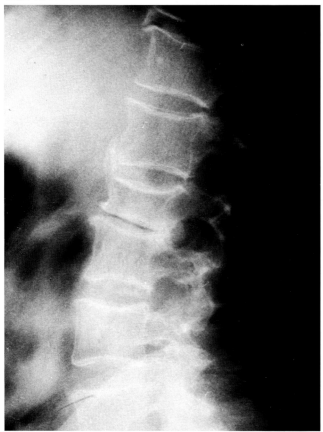

56 45 year-old male with backache after carrying heavy weights. Fell out of a tree 10 years previously.

55 Butterfly vertebra

Median fissure of vertebral body T10: anterior rhachischisis (arrow).

The butterfly vertebra is a congenital abnormality without clinical importance. This malformation occurs much more rarely than the non-closure of the neural arch (spina bifida).

56 Traumatic vertebral collapse - secondary spondylosis

Compressed fracture of vertebra L2 (1), disc narrowing and osteophyte formation (2), vacuum phenomenon (3), anterior spondylosis (4).

A traumatic vertebral collapse has to be differentiated from collapse associated with generalised osteoporosis. In primary osteoporosis, several vertebrae are affected and there is as a rule very little or no associated disc lesion or spondylosis.

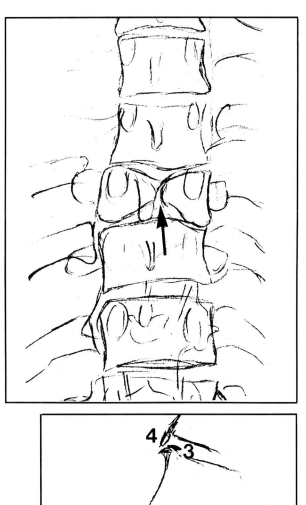

57

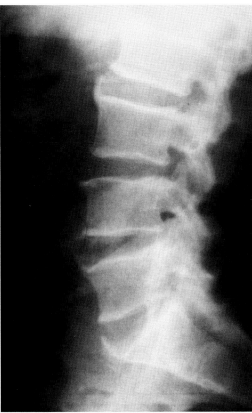

57 50 year-old male with a past history of Achilles tendinitis, right sternoclavicular arthritis and periods of backache at rest.

58

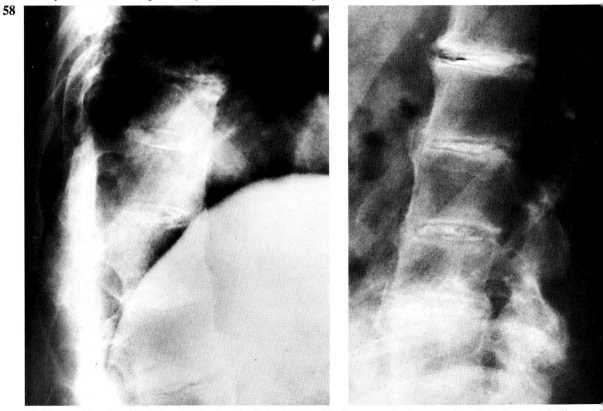

58 65 year-old male with obvious kyphosis and pain in the hips. Has been examined several times for 'glycosuria'. The test f
increased glycaemia has always been negative.

7 Ankylosing spondylitis

scending calcification of ligaments without disc arrowing (Romanus' sign).

the early stages the diagnosis of ankylosing spondylitis depends above all on the history of an flammatory type backache (pain in the second art of the night and in the morning), and associated conditions such as iritis, Achilles tendinitis and oligoarthritis. Discontinuous ligamentous alcification, either ascending or descending, sible on radiography, can help to distinguish a lvispondylitis from disc pathology with ondylosis.

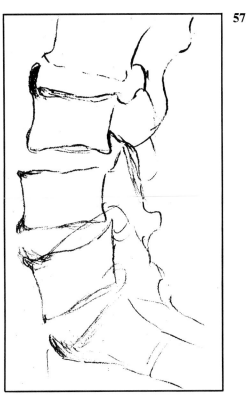

57

8 Ochronosis – alcaptonuria

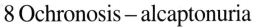

arrowed disc with calcification (1), anterior teophytosis (2), intervertebral bony bridges).

lcaptonuria is a rare hereditary recessive alady due to the total absence of the enzyme omogentisic acid oxydase. As a result of this eficiency there is an accumulation of omogentisic acid, a normal intermediate substance in the metabolism of phenylalanine and rosine.

omogentisic acid is excreted in the urine and on anding becomes black due to alkalinisation and xydation, hence the suspicion of glycosuria. In e body, homogentisic acid is retained above all cartilage and intervertebral discs, resulting in a ogressive arthropathy. Clinically the spondylo-s of alcaptonuria can resemble ankylosing spon-ylitis very closely.

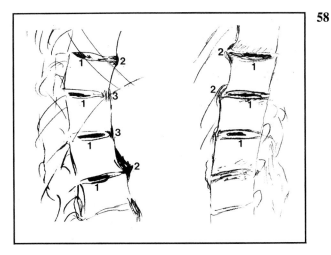

58

59

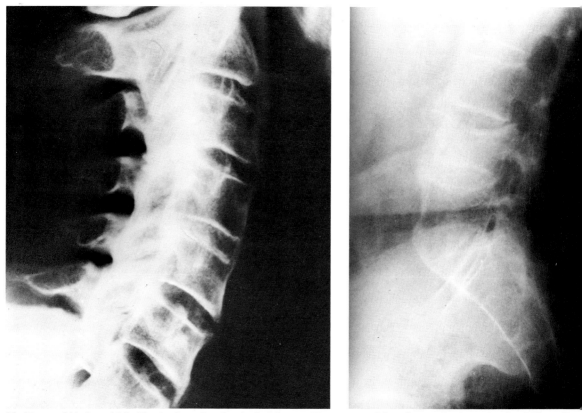

59 47 year-old baker with bad backache and neck pain for 20 years. He now complains of severe lumbar pain after falling off a barstool.

60

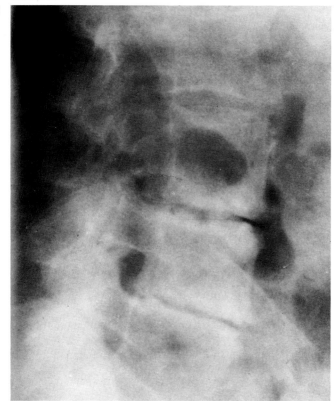

60 60 year-old female with debilitating polyarthritis for 10 years and increasing backache even at rest.

9 Ankylosing spondylitis

alcification of intervertebral ligaments (1), an-
losis of all apophyseal joints (2), fracture of L4
ith disruption of calcified ligament (3), post-
ior displacement of L4 (4), depression of L5
per surface (5).

nal stage of ankylosing spondylitis or Bech-
rew's disease, sometimes also called Marie-
rümpel's disease or pelvispondylitis ossificans.
nce the ankylosis is complete the disease causes
w complaints apart from functional restriction
tiffness). On account of the rigidity and im-
obility the subject becomes more prone to frac-
res. Most cases of ankylosing spondylitis do not
vance to this stage. It is wrong to consider only
kylosing spondylitis when radiography reveals
amboo spine.

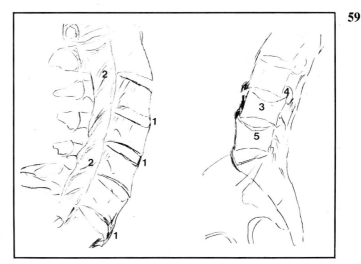

59

0 Rheumatoid spondylodiscitis

bvious disc space narrowing L3-L4, L4-L5 (1),
egular erosion of vertebral plane surfaces (2),
d sclerosis (3).

esides the well-known abnormalities of the cer-
cal spine in rheumatoid arthritis, one also sees
om time to time anomalies due to spondylo-
scitis in the lumbar spine.

milar pictures should make one think of a septic
scitis as well. In the case of septic discitis, as
so in tuberculous discitis, a single disc is usually
fected.

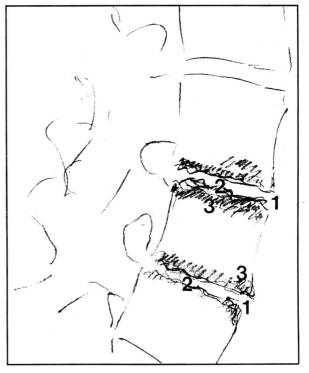

60

61

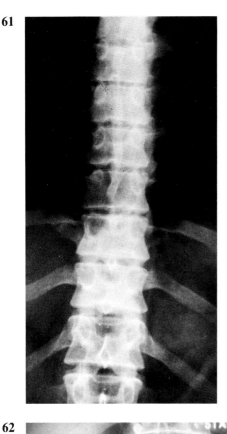

61 30 year-old commercial traveller with muscular weakness of the legs and walking difficulties for 4 weeks. Upper motor neurone signs in both lower limbs.

62

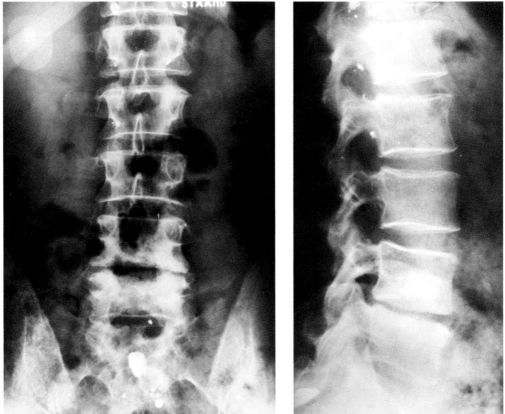

62 55 year-old miner with 8 months history of low lumbar backache radiating to the front of the thighs, and a slight temperature. He had laminectomy L4-L5. Sputum examination showed acid fast bacilli.

61 Hodgkin's disease

Osteolysis of right pedicle T9 (1), decalcification of lower part of T6 (2).

The vertebral column may be the first and only site of a lymphoma. Every bony lesion should therefore be assessed very carefully. Osteolysis or osteosclerosis of a pedicle, or of one vertebra, is pathognomonic of a malignant process, lymphoma or metastasis.

After decompression laminectomy this patient received radiotherapy. Ten years later, he is still symptom free and does heavy work. This example argues the case for early diagnosis and treatment.

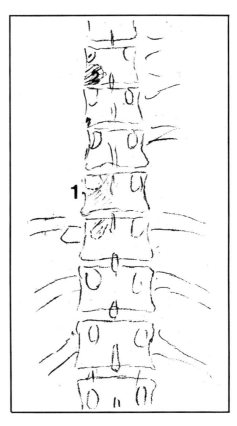

61

62 Tuberculous discitis

Overall narrowing of disc (1), central erosion of adjacent vertebral bodies (2), commencing sclerotic reactions (3), lipiodol remains (4), results of laminectomy (5).

The correct diagnosis of the cause of low backache can be difficult and rests mainly on accurate history taking and clinical examination. Special investigations should then be carried out for the purpose of confirming or refuting the clinical supposition.

From the history of the pain, one can already deduce whether it is due to an inflammatory or to a degenerative process. With an inflammatory cause the pain occurs mainly at night and in the morning, while with a degenerative lesion pain rather occurs in the evening and after weight bearing.

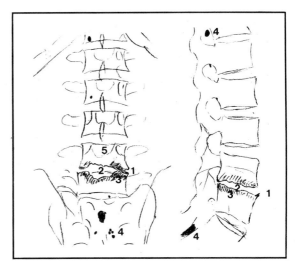

62

63

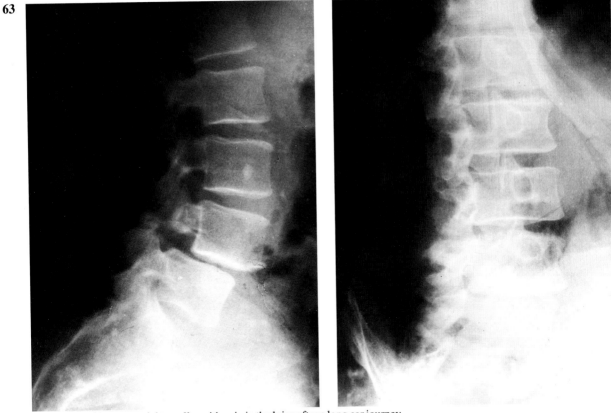

63 30 year-old commercial traveller with pain in the loins after a long car journey.

64

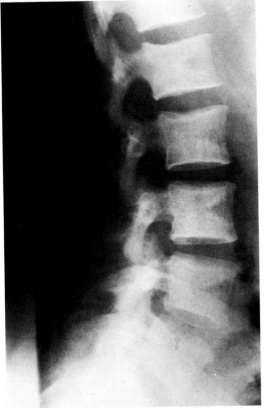

64 58 year-old charwoman with haemolytic anaemia based on an autoimmune reaction.

3 Spondylolysis – spondylolisthesis – osteopoikilosis

[ab]sence of the posterior arch of L4 (1), with [for]ward slipping of L4 (2) together with the whole [ver]tebral column above it, disc space narrowing [L4]-L5 (3), areas of sclerosis (4).

[Sp]ondylolysis occurs principally at the 3rd to 5th [lum]bar neural arch. For a long time this abnor-[ma]lity was regarded as a congenital non-fusion. [Se]rial photographs of the same patient over a [pe]riod of time now rather points to stress fracture. [On]ce the listhesis is established a secondary disc [de]generation ensues which perpetuates the [fra]cture.

[Po]ssible causes of the stress are: weight lifting, [flo]or polishing, ballet dancing, repeated falls in [chi]ldren learning to walk, weakened bone as in [Pa]get's disease, osteopetrosis, osteopoikilosis.

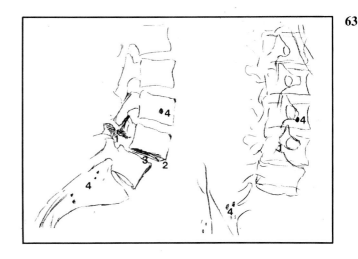

63

4 Myelosclerosis

[Ge]neralised denseness of bone structure with [spa]ring of a ventral wedge-shaped part of the [ver]tebral body.

[In] chronic myeloproliferative diseases with ex-[tra]medullary haematopoiesis, a myelosclerosis [m]ay occur, especially in old people.

[Th]e radiological picture strongly resembles that [of] osteopetrosis or Albers-Schönberg disease, [al]so called marble bone disease or osteosclerosis [fr]agilis generalisata. Most people with this her-[ed]itary disease do not live long and break their [bo]nes easily. Biochemical parameters of calcium [m]etabolism are normal.

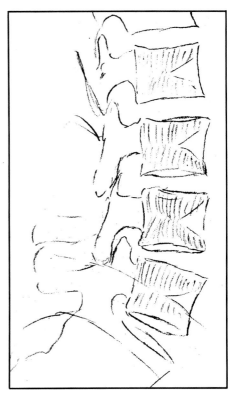

64

65

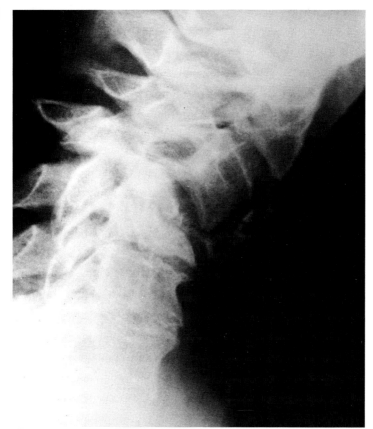

65 75 year-old male with neck pain radiating to the shoulder; has had physiotherapy for 1 year.

66

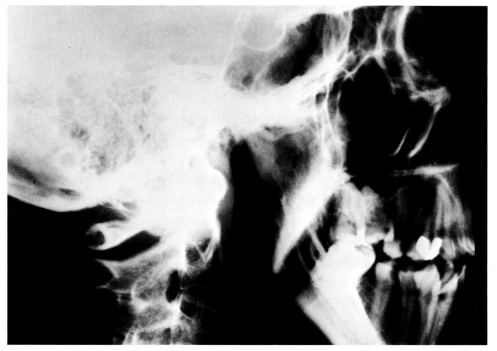

66 23 year-old employee with periodic neck and back pain, specially at night and in the morning, for 5 years. Now has very limited neck movements.

65 Tuberculous spondylodiscitis

Disc space narrowing C4-C5 (1), irregular plane surfaces (2), resorption of vertebral body C4 (3), angulation.

Although tuberculous sponylodiscitis or Pott's disease has become rare, one should remain on the lookout for it, especially in the older generations and in coloured patients.

Treatment of symptoms without a diagnosis is always dangerous. Regular review is indicated in rheumatic disorders. For tuberculous spondylodiscitis medicinal treatment is generally sufficient. In this case a stabilising procedure was necessary.

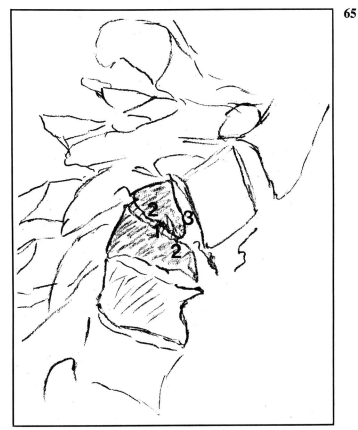

65

66 Ankylosing spondylitis

Ankylosis of the apophyseal joints (1).

Ankylosis of the cervical apophyseal joints occurs in juvenile rheumatoid arthritis and in ankylosing spondylitis. A simple congenital fusion of a single joint can also occur. It has been observed for a long time that cases of juvenile rheumatoid arthritis appear in the families of patients with ankylosing spondylitis. A key to this familial link lies in the increased frequency of occurrence of HLA antigen B27 in these patients and their close relatives.

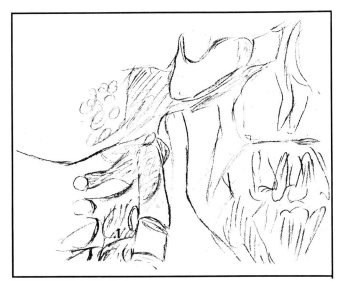

66

67

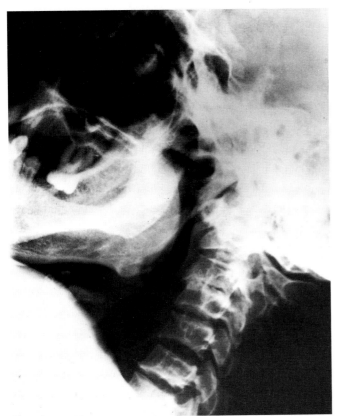

67 50 year-old male with debilitating polyarthritis and marked restriction of movement of the neck, which appears shortened.

68

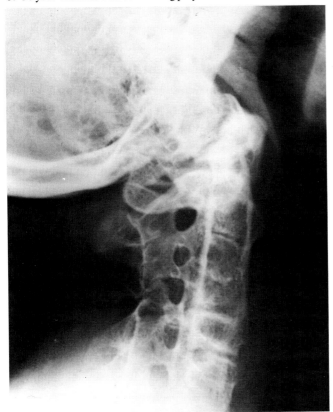

68 13 year-old boy with a tilt of the head, no contracture of the sternocleidomastoid, and elevation of the right shoulder.

67 Rheumatoid arthritis – basilar impression – spondylodiscitis

The dens extends more than 5mm above McGregor's plane (1), mild atlantoaxial subluxation (2), subluxation C3-C4 (3), discitis and erosion of plane surfaces C3-C4 and C6-C7 (4), erosive arthritis apophyseal joint C6-C7 (5).

In rheumatoid arthritis serious lesions often develop in the vertebral column, which may give rise to neurological complications such as quadriparesis and quadriplegia. Warning symptoms of a transverse lesion are shooting pains with spontaneous movements in the arms and legs.

The articular surfaces are eroded by the rheumatoid process with resulting laxity of ligaments and subluxation.

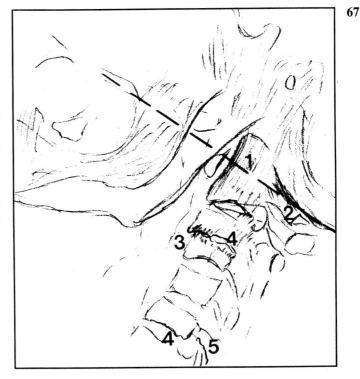

67

68 Klippel-Feil syndrome with Sprengel's deformity

Fusion of vertebrae C2-C3 (1), C5-C6 (2), fusion of apophyseal joints (3), calcified ligamentous ridges anteriorly (4).

Fusion of the greater part of the cervical spine into one block is characteristic of the Klippel-Feil syndrome. This abnormality is often accompanied by a raised shoulder. The scapula has failed to descend from its embryonic position; this congenital abnormality is called Sprengel's deformity.

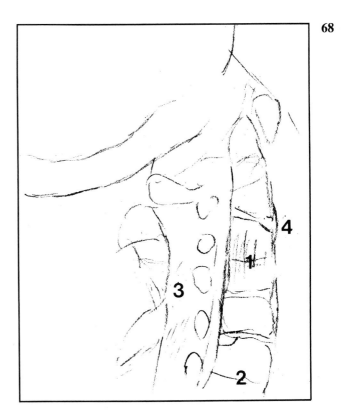

68

69

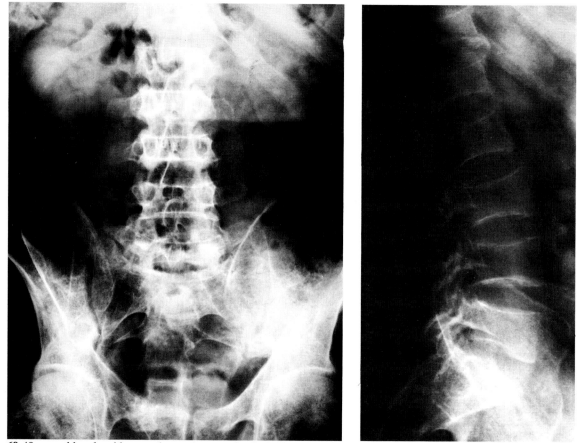

69 40 year-old male with muscular weakness and a duck-like gait for a few years; swelling of right knee. Normal growth and development in youth.

70

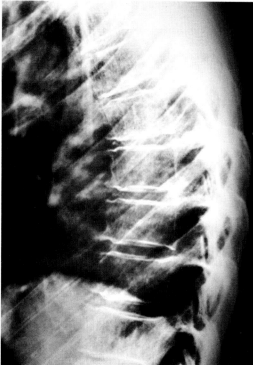

70 40 year-old female complaining of headaches and, for the past few years, thick, heavy hands and feet.

69 Osteomalacia in phosphorus diabetes

Hazy bone structure, platyspondylosis, enlarged disc spaces, deformed neck of femur with pseudofracture (1), also pseudofracture of the superior pubic ramus (2), and ribs (3).

Phosphorus diabetes is characterised by a constantly low level of serum phosphorus due to its loss by urinary excretion, the blood calcium level remaining normal. Vitamin D therapy together with phosphorus by mouth will alleviate the muscular weakness and the bone lesions. Usually very large doses of vitamin D are required hence the name vitamin D resistant rickets.

The causes of phosphorus depletion are:
– Hereditary renal tubular defects,
familial hypophosphataemia
cystinosis (De Toni-Debré-Fanconi syndrome).
– Acquired renal tubular defects,
hereditary tyrosinaemia
Wilson's disease
neurofibromatosis
mesenchymal tumour.
– Malabsorption of phosphorus due to chronic

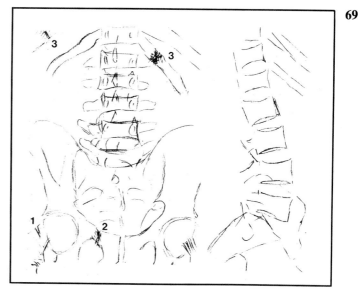

69

administration of aluminium hydroxide antacids.

Our patient had a phosphorus diabetes secondary to a mesenchymal tumour of the knee.

70 Acromegaly

Appositional bone (1) and osteophytosis (2) on the fronts of the thoracic vertebrae.

Acromegaly produces typical deformities in the vertebral column especially in the thoracic region. Anterior hypertrophy of the vertebral bodies becomes manifest as well as a tendency to early spondylosis. Increase in volume gives the vertebra the appearance of a coarse-mesh osteoporosis.

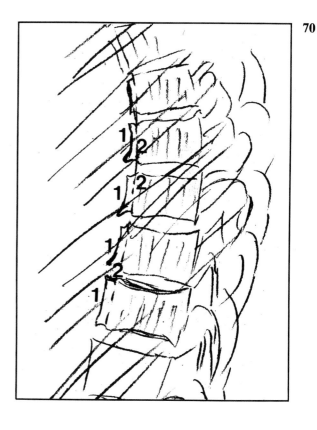

70

71

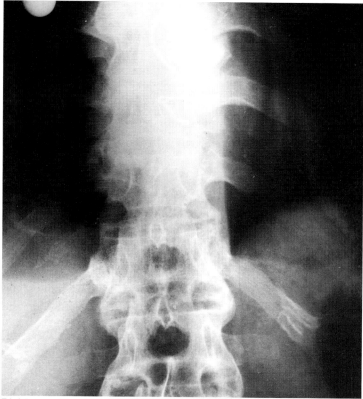

71 35 year-old employee complaining of loin pain. A cardiac murmur was discovered in the course of a medical examination for l assurance. Two years later an artificial valve was inserted for aortic incompetence. During his military service he suffered a bout sciatica.

72

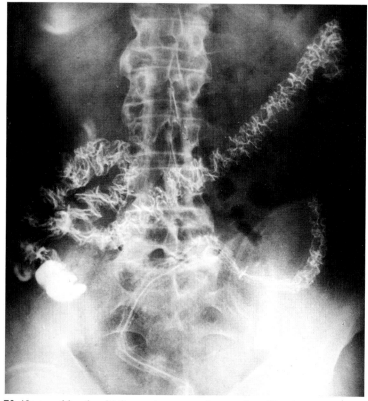

72 40 year-old male with frequent mucopurulent stools and low backache.

71 Ankylosing spondylitis

Syndesmophytes (1), artificial valve (2).

Aortic valvular disease occurs in 1 to 4 per cent of patients with ankylosing spondylitis, usually in the form of aortic incompetence. Conduction anomalies are present in 8 per cent of cases. A quarter of the patients with spondylitis are troubled with iritis, often before the appearance of back trouble.

In its typical form ankylosing spondylitis occurs 8 times more frequently in males than in females. However, abortive cases of inflammatory back-ache often occur in women, usually without radiological signs. The pelvispondylitic diathesis is genetic, related to the presence of human leucocyte antigen (HLA) B27. 80 per cent of spondylitis patients are HLA B27 positive, but only 7 per cent of the normal population.

72 Pelvispondylitis associated with ulcerative colitis

Bilateral sacroiliitis (1), lower third of sacroiliac joints hazy and eroded, showing sclerotic reaction and syndesmophytes (2). Rectocolitis: abnormal pattern of intestinal mucosa, loss of hacculations (3).

About 20 per cent of patients with ulcerative colitis and 5 per cent of those with regional ileitis (Crohn's disease) develop an associated arthritis. Two clinical patterns are distinguished — peripheral arthritis on the one hand and pelvispondylitis on the other. The abnormalities of pelvispondylitis are often indistinguishable from ankylosing spondylitis.

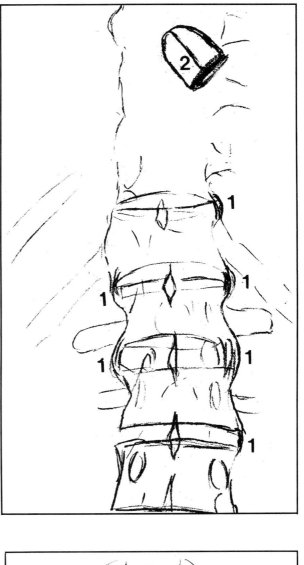

71

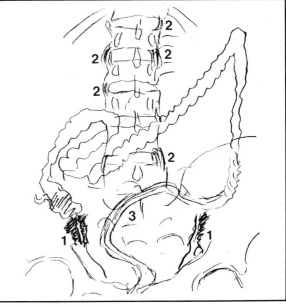

72

73

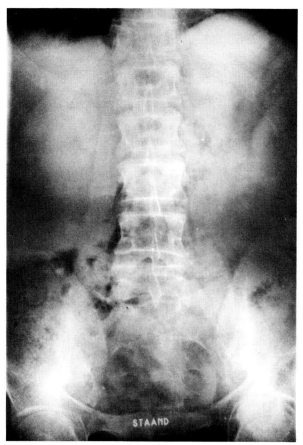

73 50 year-old male with psoriasis and arthritis, treated for years with low doses of corticosteroids.

74

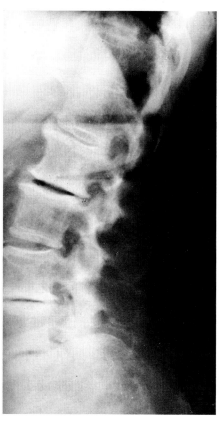

74 65 year-old housewife with intermittent backache for many years particularly after heavy work. Now and then severe attacks of lumbar pain.

3 Psoriatic spondylitis cortisone osteoporosis

rasyndesmophyte to the left of L2-L3 (1), hazy
ght and left sacroiliac joints (2), flattening of
.2 and L5 (3), aseptic necrosis of head of left
mur with joint space diminution (4).

though corticosteroids have antiphlogistic and
algesic effects on inflammatory rheumatism,
ey are not indicated in most chronic rheumatic
nditions, even in low dosage. The side effects
.e osteoporosis with vertebral collapse, aseptic
crosis of the head of the femur and cataract, are
eversible and aggravate the original handicap
r which they are given.

4 Trophostatic syndrome

creased lumbar lordosis (1), disc degeneration
ith vacuum phenomenon (2), apophyseal
thropathy (3), spondylolisthesis (4), postero-
thesis (5), interspinous arthropathy (Baas-
up's disease) (6), osteophytosis (7).

postclimacteric women, a syndrome often
curs which is characterised clinically by back-
he of the type due to overloading, lumbar
perlordosis, thoracic kyphosis, weak abdo-
inal muscles and protruding abdomen.
adiologically there are signs of degenerative
sc disease and its sequelae. Such women have
id either multiple pregnancies or a number of
dominal operations like cholecystectomy or
sterectomy.

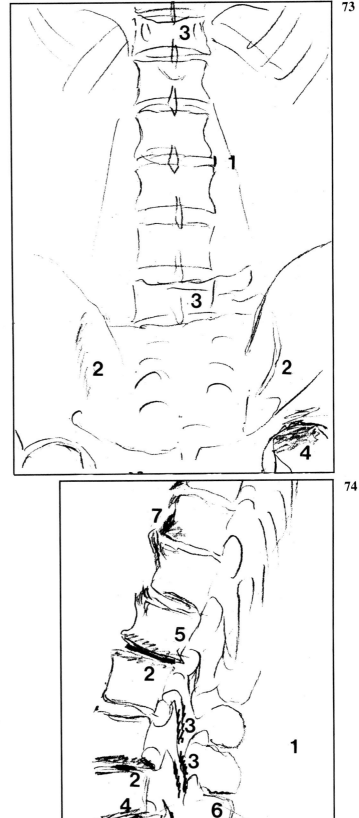

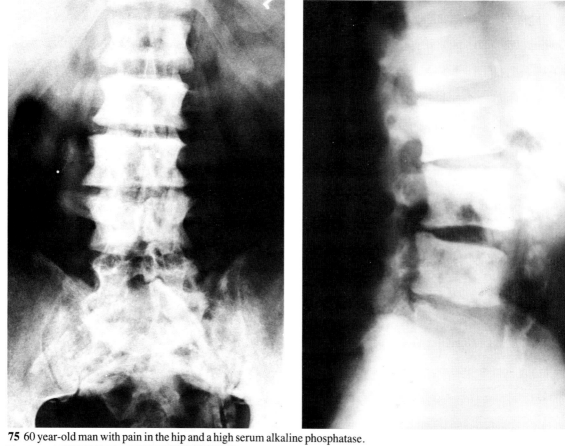

75 60 year-old man with pain in the hip and a high serum alkaline phosphatase.

76

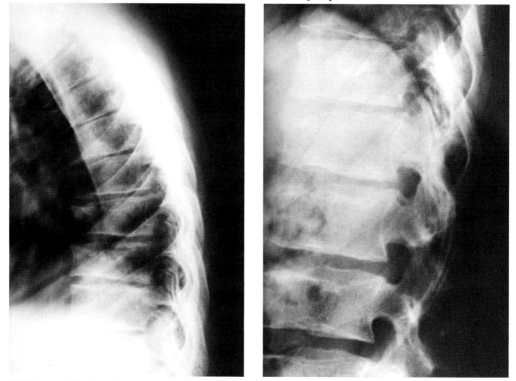

76 31 year-old miner with pain in his knees and stiffness of the hips after exertion. Short stature with kyphosis. Can still walk metres with crutches. One brother has similar complaints.

5 Paget's disease

...neven density with transverse and anteroposter-...r expansion of L2, L3 and L4 compared with L1 ...d L5 (arrows). Uneven dense and trabecular ...ucture of left ilium.

...e bone lesions of Paget's disease develop in 3 ...ges: the first stage is no more than osteolysis ...th sometimes the collapse of a vertebra. The ...cond stage shows new bone formation of the ...rtex, accounting for the expansion, sclerosis ...d picture-frame image. The third stage is a ...mbination of osteolysis and osteosclerosis with ...sorderly alteration of bone architecture. The ...sions are generally asymptomatic unless they ...use compression of a neighbouring nerve or ...less a joint, usually the hip or knee, is com-...omised.

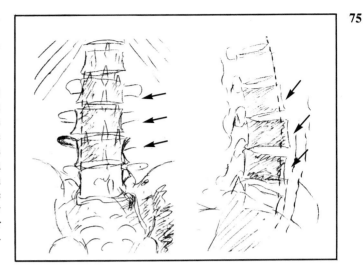

6 Tardive form of spondyloepiphyseal dysplasia

...ide, flat vertebral bodies (platyspondylosis) ...), cuneiform compression (2), and irregular ...ane surfaces (3) with anterior osteophytosis (4).

...here are various types of spondyloepiphyseal ...ysplasia, all characterised by a small stature ...anism), flat, irregular vertebrae (platyspondyl-...m) and involvement of the proximal joints with ...arly secondary arthropathy of hips and shoul-...ers. The face and skull are normal. The different ...pes are classified according to the age of onset of ...bnormalities and the mode of inheritance.

...ailey's classification:
. Congenital spondyloepiphyseal dysplasia
. Pseudoachondroplasia (type I-IV)
. Pseudo Morquio's syndrome (type I-IV)
. Tardive spondyloepiphyseal dysplasia:
   a. X-linked
   b. Brachyraphia
   c. Brachyolmia.

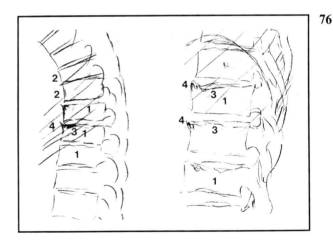

77

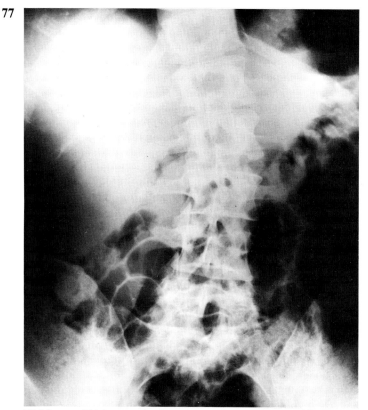

77 24 year-old labourer who from time to time sprains an ankle. He wears glasses and is very tall (1.80m), with an arm span 1.90m, very long fingers, genu recurvatum and a very supple spine. He can reach the ground with his wrists.

78

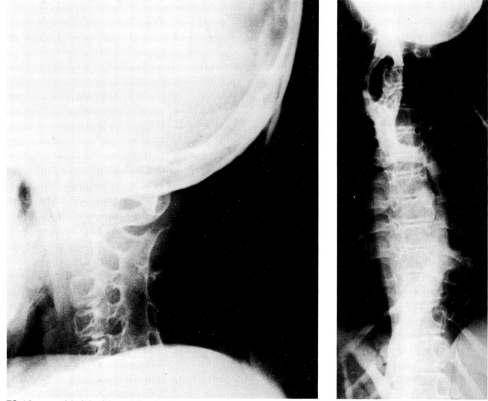

78 10 year-old girl with rapidly developing contractures of hips and shoulders. Unable to walk for 6 weeks.

77 Scoliosis with Marfan's syndrome

Marfan's syndrome, also known as arachnodactyly (spider fingers), is a hereditary connective tissue disorder characterised by eye, bone and cardiovascular abnormalities. The most important defect of the eye is ectopia lentis and of the cardiovascular system, aneurysm of the ascending aorta. The particular skeletal anomaly is the extraordinary length of the extremities. Abnormal laxity of the joints may lead to frequent sprains or dislocations.

In many cases scoliosis (arrow), probably due to joint weakness, is a grave problem. Hypermobility of the joints occurs also in various forms of Ehlers-Danlos syndrome, osteogenesis imperfecta and in familial hypermobility syndrome.

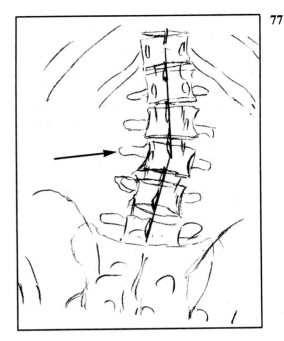

77

78 Progressive myositis ossificans

Fusion of all apophyseal joints (1), ossification of the attachments of neck muscles (2), sternocleidomastoid (3), back and thorax muscles (4).

Progressive myositis ossificans is a rare congenital disorder of the mesodermal tissues which may manifest at any age between birth and puberty. Ectopic bone develops in the intermuscular septa, followed by extension into the muscles. Ankylosis of neighbouring joints may occur.

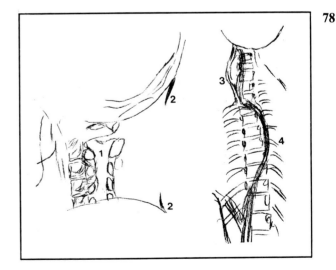

78

79

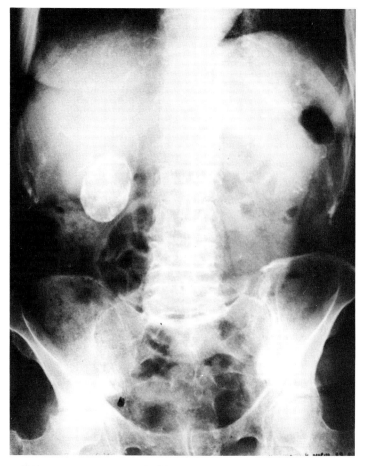

79 70 year-old lady with increasing pain in the right hip for 5 months; gradual shortening of stature from 1.67m to 1.52m. She is being treated for a hyperlipidaemia.

80

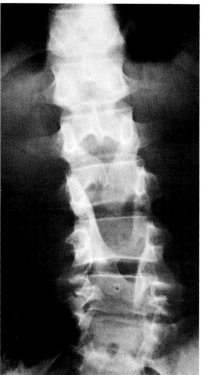

80 15 year-old schoolgirl with bilateral talipes equinovarus.

9 Postmenopausal axial osteoporosis – aseptic necrosis of head of femur

ultiple depressions of vertebrae T12, L2, L3, 4 (1), necrosis of right femoral head with partial eformity (2), porcelain gall bladder (3) calcified ostal cartilages (4).

) to 15 years after the menopause some women evelop severe osteoporosis leading to depression of vertebrae. The most obvious clinical anifestation is progressive shrinking of the stare with periods of girdle type radiation of pain. hese patients usually have no radiological signs ' arthrosis or spondylosis.

he hyperlipidaemia can be a causal factor in eptic necrosis.

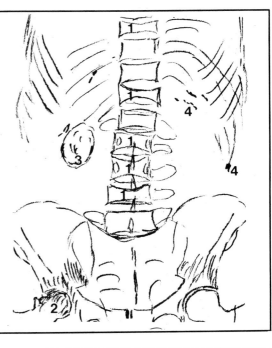

79

0 Spina bifida occulta

on-fusion of neural arches L3, L4, L5 (arrows).

onclosure of a neural arch is usually asymp-matic. Mild degrees of spina bifida of L5 and S1 re common. About 20 per cent of normal people ow such a malformation of one vertebra. Some eople with spina bifida however show a neurolo-ically induced abnormality of the lower limbs, uch as club foot or a neuropathic arthropathy due sensory disturbances.

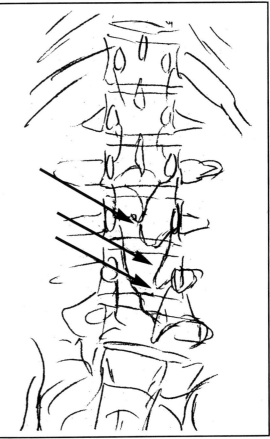

80

3: Hip and shoulder

The coxofemoral and scapulohumeral articulations present specialised anatomical constructions, adapted to functional requirements. The shoulder has to provide maximal freedom of movement in all directions and the hips are required not only to transmit the weight of the trunk to the lower limbs but also to allow for extensive mobility in many directions.

In the case of the hip, the anatomical architecture on which it operates biomechanically is of great importance, whereas with the shoulder the emphasis is on its system of suspension, seeing that there is little bony support. Since this system of suspension does not show up in the usual radiographic plates, one sees, radiographically, less pathology in the shoulder than in the hips.

These articulations being very mobile, it is possible to radiograph them in many different positions. In order to interpret a radiograph correctly it is extremely important to know the exact position, otherwise erroneous interpretations may result. As in the case of other joints, left-right comparison is very useful in order to recognise anatomical variations and to disclose early signs of disease.

It should be stressed that radiography of the skeleton reveals on the whole late changes. The history and clinical examination remain the basis of a good diagnosis.

There is a tendency to attribute pain in the region of the shoulder girdle to cervical arthrosis and for all discomfort around the hip to be called coxarthrosis. Radiological diagnosis of hip joint disease is not enough; the cause should always be sought in order to determine whether the abnormality is primary or secondary.

Secondary hip joint disease can arise in many conditions as the following radiographs bring out.

81

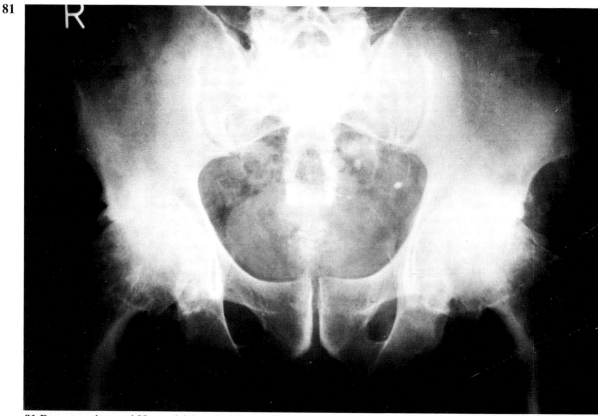

81 Factory worker aged 55 complaining of pain in the right knee for 5 years. He weighs 109kg and is 1.79m tall.

82

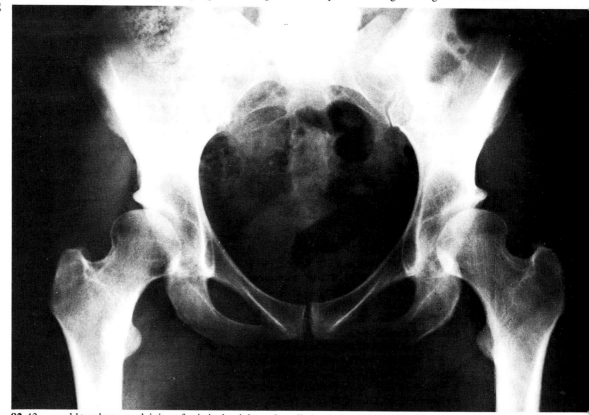

82 43 year-old teacher complaining of pain in the right groin radiating to the right knee, which started after a long walk.

81 Primary coxarthrosis

Irregular narrowing of the superolateral part of the hip joint space both right and left (1), with neighbouring subchondral sclerosis (2), osteophytosis along the articular margin (3) and formation of an osteophytic shelf below (4).

Among the osteoarthroses, that of the hip is the most debilitating. 50 per cent of coxarthroses occur within the framework of a polyarthrosis. The rest are the outcome of anatomical changes, abnormalities of the pelvis, Paget's disease, coxitis, trauma, and aseptic necrosis. At the stage when narrowing of the joint space is detectable on radiography, persistent pain has set in. Osteophyte formation confined to the articular margin hardly causes any pain.

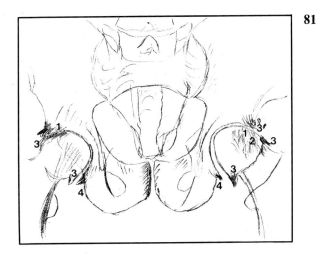

81

82 Dysplasia of the hip with secondary coxarthrosis

Slight narrowing of the right hip joint space (1), malformation of the acetabular roof with a slope of 25 degrees (normal = 10 degrees) (2), coxa valga with cervicodiaphyseal angle 145 degrees (normal = 135 degrees) (3), inadequate roofing over femoral heads (4).

Normally the roof of the acetabulum is nearly horizontal and overhangs the head of the femur almost completely. Dysplasia of the hip occurs more commonly in females than in males and is often hereditary and familial. The malformation is characterised by an underdevelopment of the roof of the acetabulum anteriorly and laterally with consequent insufficient covering of the head of the femur. Often there is at the same time a coxa valga and hyperanteversion of the neck of the femur. The anomaly presents uni- or bilaterally with equal frequency.

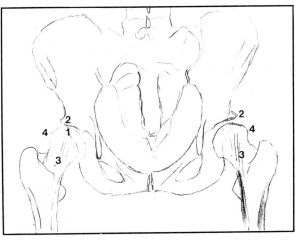

82

83

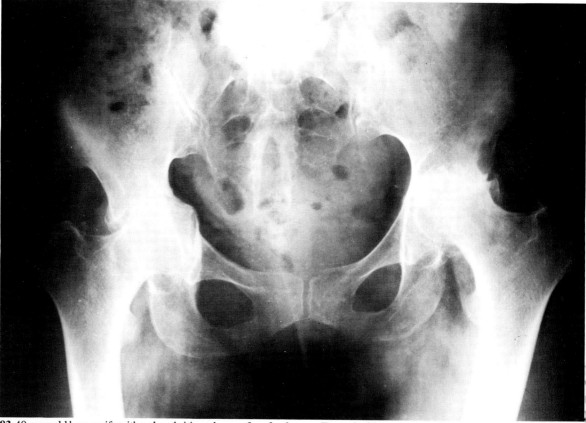

83 40 year-old housewife with polyarthritis and moon face for 6 years. Treated with corticosteroids.

84

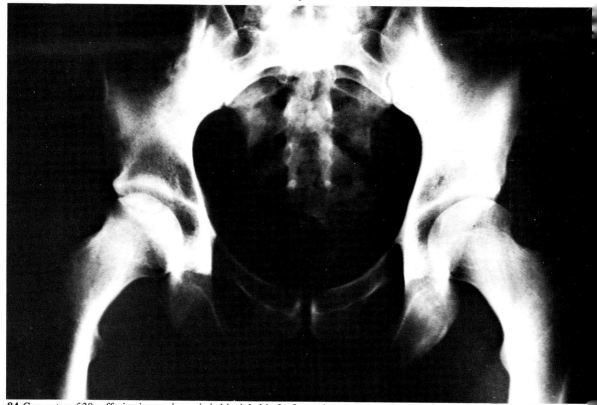

84 Carpenter of 38 suffering increasing pain in his right hip for 3 months, aggravated by walking. The pain appeared suddenly.

3 Rheumatic coxitis – cortisone hip

eneral narrowing of the joint space (1) with
rotrusion (2) more marked on the right. Necrosis
f the head of the femur on the left (3), neighbour-
g osteosclerosis (4).

rheumatoid arthritis, the hip lesion presents the
cture of a coxitis, to be distinguished from a
xarthrosis by the generalised narrowing of the
int space, periarticular osteoporosis and the
sence of osteophytic reaction. Note that the use
corticosteroids favours the tendency for protru-
on and development of aseptic necrosis.

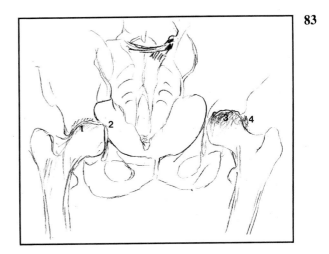

83

4 Idiopathic aseptic necrosis of the femoral head (Chandler's disease)

eparation of the necrosed segment (1), with
djacent sclerosis (2).

diopathic aseptic necrosis of the head of the
emur is more common in males than in females
nd appears around the age of 40-60 years. There
s often an associated disorder of fat metabolism
nd an elevated serum uric acid level. The disease
requently accompanies excessive alcohol in-
ake. The lesion is commonly bilateral. At the
nset, during the first weeks and up to two months
ne cannot reveal any radiological changes. Dur-
ng this period a scintiscan of the skeleton shows
n abnormal concentration of isotopes in the
ffected part. Necrosis of the head of the femur
ccurs with relatively greater frequency in a num-
er of systemic disorders like rheumatoid arthritis
nd lupus erythematosis disseminatus and also
fter prolonged administration of corticosteroids.
he idiopathic form is also called Chandler's
isease.

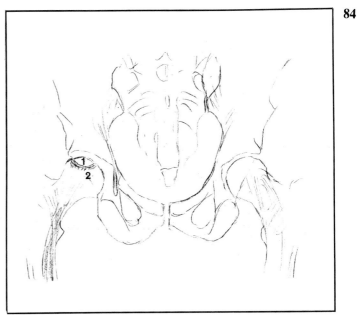

84

85

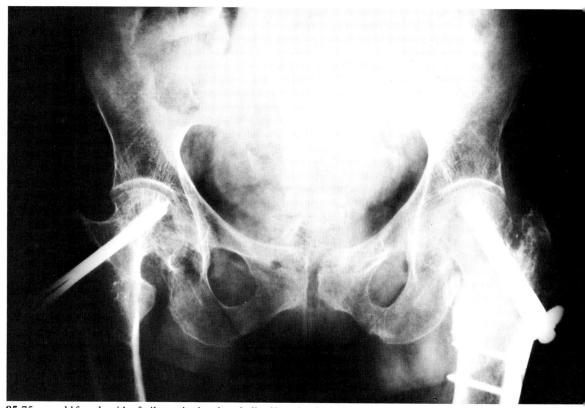

85 75 year-old female with a frail constitution, hospitalised in an institution for chronic diseases; fracture of the right neck of femur at the age of 68, intertrochanteric fracture at 72, in both instances due to a slight fall.

86

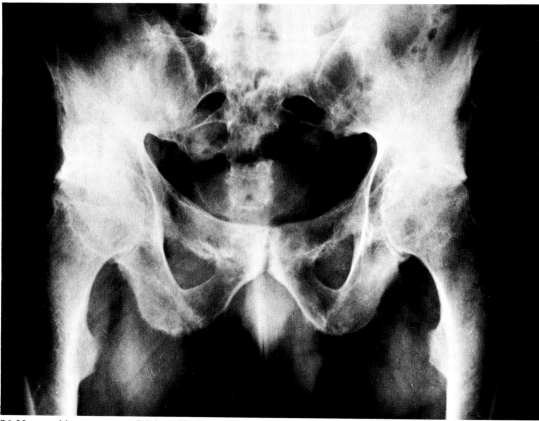

86 33 year-old postman complaining of backache for 8 years. At present he has pain on walking, particularly in the morning and after sitting for a long period.

5 Fracture of the neck of the femur – osteoporosis

mith-Petersen pin on the right (1) and Mac-
aughlin pin and plate on the left (2).

fracture of the neck of the femur caused by
inimal trauma is generally regarded as the result
´ a generalised osteoporosis promoted by in-
easing decalcification with age. Neck of femur
actures occur with increasing frequency after
e age of 60, more so in women than in men.
hese fractures also occur more often in white
an in non-white subjects.

every case of fractured neck of femur an
ssociated vitamin D deficiency should be ex-
uded. With an osteoporosis the biochemical
arameters of calcium metabolism are normal
hile they are altered in osteomalacia. In cases
ith osteoporosis the fractures heal well.

onsidering the advanced age of a patient with a
actured neck of the femur, one usually decides

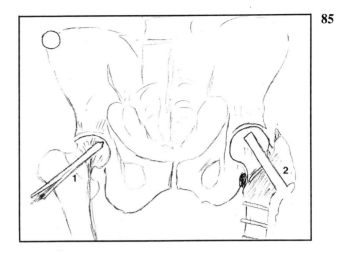

85

on surgical fixation to avoid the unfavourable
effects of prolonged immobilisation. A Moore's
prosthesis is sometimes preferred because pin-
ning may lead to necrosis of the head of the femur.

6 Ankylosing spondylitis

omplete IVth degree fusion of the sacroiliac
ints (1), bilateral coxitis (2) with uniform nar-
wing of the joint space, absence of osteophyte
rmation, pubic osteitis (3), irregular contour of
e lesser trochanter (4) and ischium (5), syndes-
ophytes (6).

he radiological signs of ankylosing spondylitis
re characteristic but only appear long after the
rst signs manifest clinically. Sometimes the
atient may experience lumbosacral pain for
ears during the night as well as in the daytime,
ithout a definite sacroiliac arthritis being de-
onstrable radiologically.

he first radiological signs of sacroiliac arthritis
re: blurred articular margins, especially those of
e lower one-third, widened joint space, small
rosions, and later, bony bridges.

esides the involvement of the sacroiliac joints
nd the vertebral column, the hips are also
ffected (coxitis) in a number of cases. One often

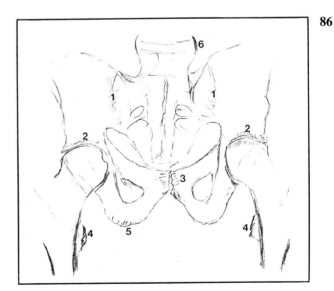

86

sees erosive lesions at the sites of attachment of
tendons and aponeuroses to the pelvis, especially
the iliac crest, the pubic rami and the lesser
trochanter.

87

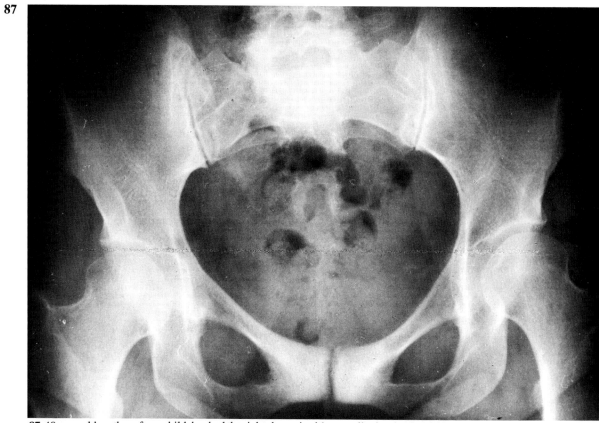

87 40 year-old mother of one child; has had the right shoe raised 1 cm to alleviate her headache.

88

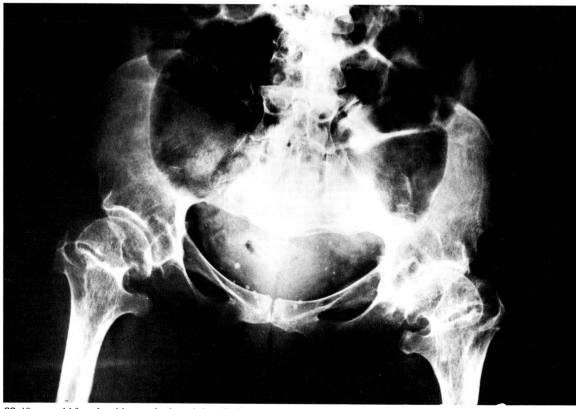

88 40 year-old female with paraplegia and short limbs.

87 Pubic osteitis

ndistinct and irregular outline of the symphysis pubis (1), sclerosis of the neighbouring bone (2), aulty measurement of length of lower limbs (3) due to tilting of pelvis (4).

Although the osteitis of the symphysis pubis in this case was identified by chance on radiography, it can cause pain in the pubic region. The pain is aggravated by walking or standing and diminishes with rest. The discomfort is accentuated by contraction of the adductor muscles. The complaint often results from urological or obstetical manoeuvres. A purulent or chronic osteitis should be excluded. The condition usually resolves after a few weeks or months but may persist or a prolonged period.

The practice of drawing a conclusion regarding the difference in length of the limbs on pelvic radiographs is not to be recommended. This method gives too many wrong results to be used as the basis for treatment.

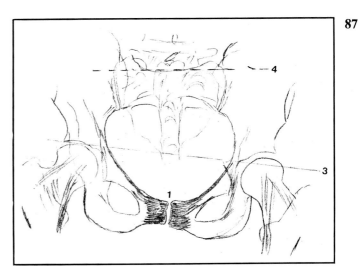

87

88 Achondroplasia

Deformity of the proximal end of the femur; abnormally prominent lesser (1) and greater (2) trochanters, absence of neck of femur (3) narrow pelvic inlet (4).

Achondroplasia is the commonest form of chondroplasia (1 in 10,000 births). 15 per cent occur in parents who are also affected (autosomal dominant). In 80 per cent of cases the family history is negative, and here the genetic anomaly must therefore be the result of mutation.

The trunk is normal but the vertebral pedicles are too close together, leading to compression of the spinal cord and consequent paraplegia in some cases. The pelvic inlet is grossly narrowed and in case of pregnancy a caesarean section should be performed. Early hip arthrosis occurs as a result of altered anatomical relations.

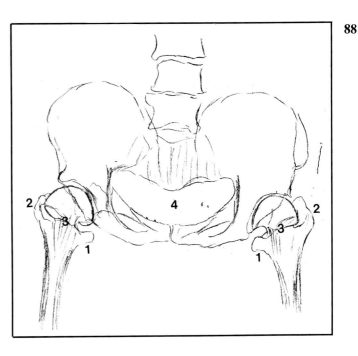

88

89

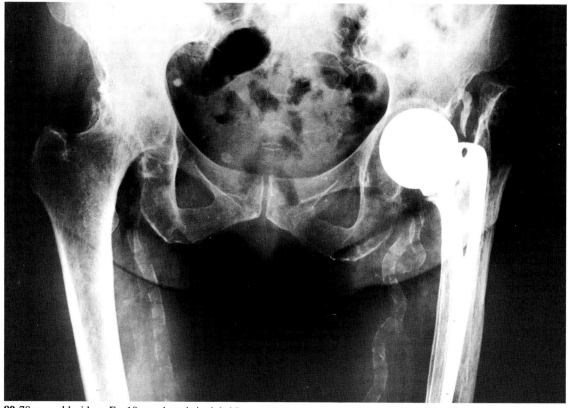

89 78 year-old widow. For 18 months pain in right hip on walking. 10 years earlier, broke the neck of her left femur in a car acciden After a Moore's prosthesis was inserted, progressive sense of instability in her left leg.

90

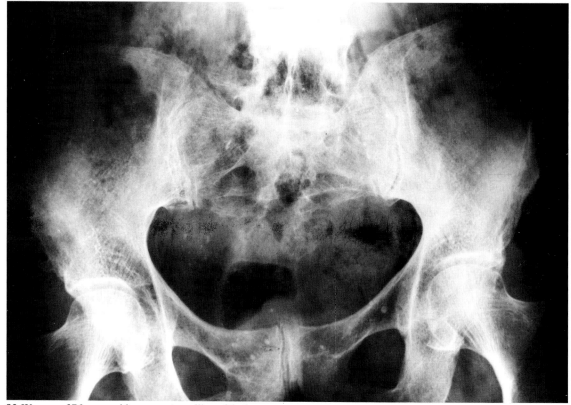

90 Woman of 76 years with recurrent swelling of the knees.

89 Coxarthrosis – loose Moore's prosthesis

Narrowing of the hip joint space on the right (1), especially above and centrally with sclerosis (2), or cyst formation (3), Moore prosthesis on the left (4), prosthesis loosened (5), periosteal reaction (6), Mönckeberg's sclerosis (7).

The loosening of a prosthesis reveals itself radiographically by a space in which the prosthesis can move, and by periosteal reaction. Note the almost complete resorption of the cortex.

The osteoarthrosis on the right is of the type that is accompanied by protrusion with pushing in of the acetabulum. Usually coxarthrosis with protrusion does not produce much pain.

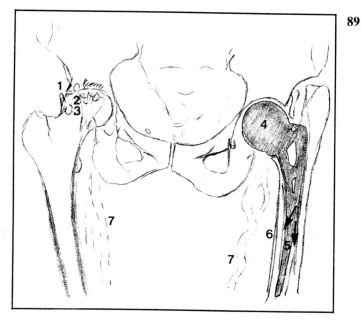

89

90 Chondrocalcinosis of the symphysis pubis

Opaque line in the fibrocartilaginous part of the pubic symphysis (arrow).

In some cases chondrocalcinosis can be totally asymptomatic, whilst in others it may cause severe joint pain with secondary arthrosis especially in the hips and knees. The disease presents most commonly at an advanced age, is sometimes familial and is often associated with other disorders such as diabetes mellitus, hyperparathyroidism or haemochromatosis.

Because of the occurrence of attacks of monoarticular arthritis due to a calcium pyrophosphate crystal synovitis, usually in the knee, the disease is also called pseudogout.

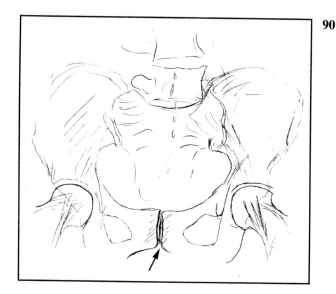

90

91

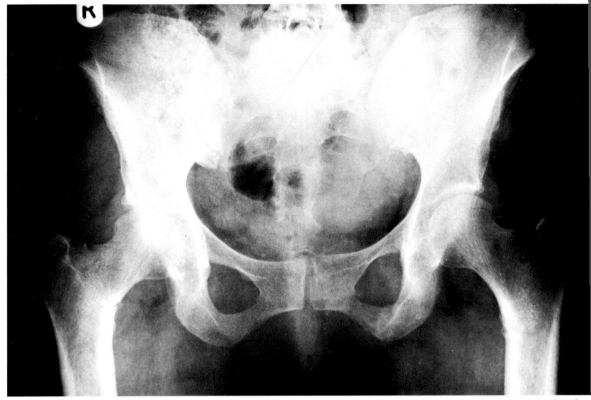

91 44 year-old female with a 3 year history of muscular weakness and increasing disability for which repeated investigations have been carried out in a neurological institute.

92

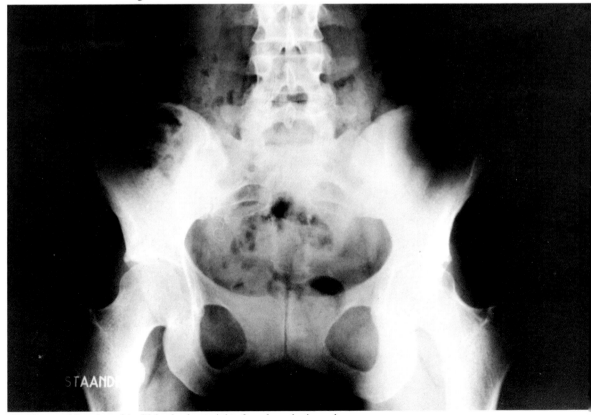

92 30 year-old mother of 4 with backache at night after a long day's work.

91 Osteomalacia in phosphorus diabetes

Pseudofracture of neck of right femur (1), of shaft of left femur (2) and of the left ischiopubic ramus (3); generally blurred appearance of bone.

One of the first clinical signs of an abnormal metabolism of vitamin D is muscular weakness, which causes a typical waddling gait. With vitamin D therapy improvement of the muscular weakness takes place as the skeletal parameters are restored in the serum as well as on radiography. Phosphorus diabetes in the adult, leading to a vitamin D resistant osteomalacia, is rare and is usually caused by renal tubular abnormality.

The radiographic picture of osteomalacia is typified by the presence of pseudofractures which always calls for investigation of the calcium metabolism. In cases of phosphorus diabetes the serum phosphorus is always low and phosphorus excretion in the urine is raised.

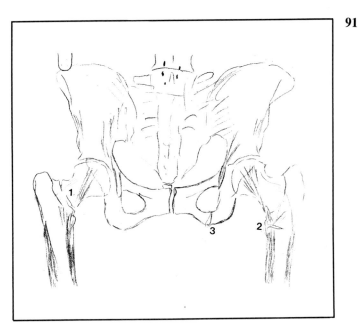

92 Osteitis condensans of the ilium

Triangular dense zone of the right ilium adjacent to lower part of sacroiliac joint (1). Sacroiliac joint space normal.

Osteitis condensans of the ilium is nearly always a chance radiological observation in women who have had multiple pregnancies. Apart from nonspecific backache, which may be confined to the lower lumbar regions, there are no clinical complaints. The radiological picture, showing sclerosis of the ilium opposite the lower part of the sacroiliac joint, may disappear completely after a time.

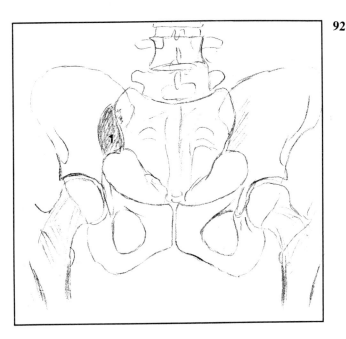

93

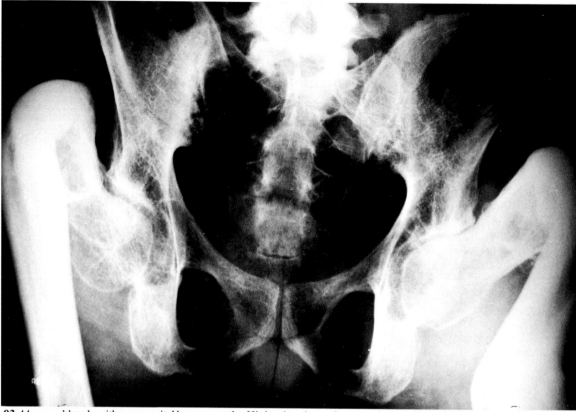

93 44 year-old male with a congenital bone anomaly. His brother shows the same abnormality, with fractures in his youth.

94

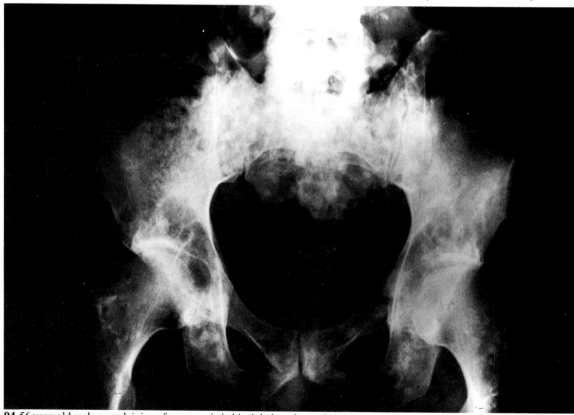

94 56 year-old male complaining of severe pain in his right leg, day and night.

93 Coxa vara associated with polycystic fibrous dysplasia

Extreme coxa vara deformity with shepherd's crook formation (1), healed fracture (2).

This disease is a fibrous tissue abnormality of unknown origin of the skeletal system which was previously also called fibrocystic disease. The medullary bone is replaced by fibrous tissue but retains bone elements. The disease may affect a small segment of bone but may also be more extensive. The pelvis, femur, skull and thorax are mainly affected. Deformities develop due to the fragility of the fibrous tissue and fractures occur with bone tissue reaction. Symptoms and deformities usually appear during the first and second decades.

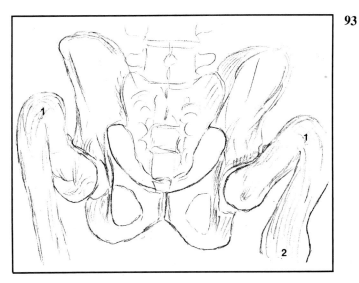

93

94 Osteoblastic metastases

Dense areas (1), unevenly distributed in the pelvis, sacrum, left transverse process of L5 (2), rarefaction of acetabulum, head and neck of femur on the right (3).

Bone pain without circadian rhythm, equally intense night and day, should always make one suspect neoplastic infiltration. In the case of osteoarthrosis, the pain appears above all on weight bearing. With an arthritis it troubles the patient mostly in the morning and in the second part of the night. Bone metastases may be silent and only discovered by chance on radiography; on the other hand they may cause symptoms while not showing up on X-ray during the first months. In this latter case, a skeletal scintiscan with technetium can be very useful and lead to an early diagnosis.

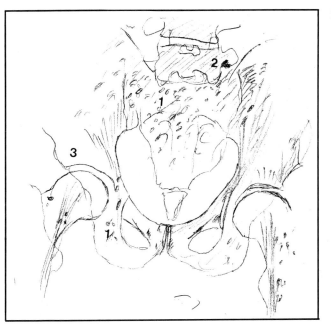

94

95

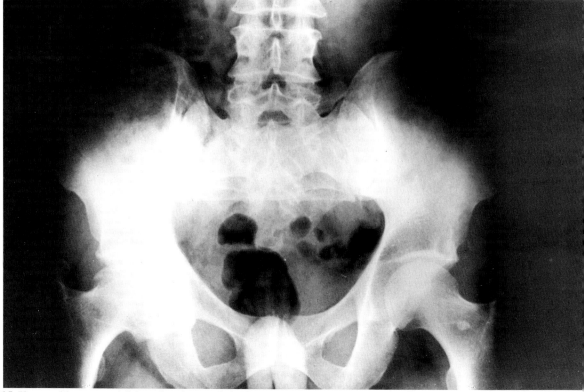

95 52 year-old man complaining of moderate pain in his right hip. Runs 20km cross country 3 times a week. At the age of 12 had a pain in his right hip for 3 weeks.

96

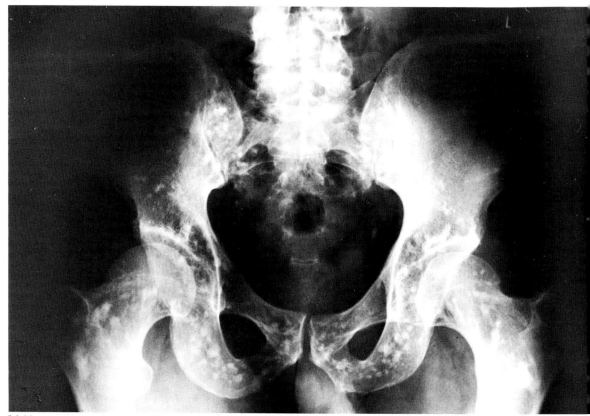

96 30 year-old commercial traveller complaining of backache after a long car journey.

95 Adolescent coxa vara

Slipped head of femur on the right (1), central joint space narrowing (2), early osteophytosis (3), dense bony island in neck of left femur (4).

Coxa vara of adolescence is a result of epiphysiolysis of the femoral head. The epiphysis of the head of the femur unites with the shaft between the ages of 16 and 19; just before uniting (between 10 and 17 years of age, with a peak at 11-13 for girls and 13-16 for boys) the head of the femur may be displaced medially and backwards.

Although the displacement is sometimes associated with an acute injury, its onset is usually surreptitious. The disorder occurs more often in boys.

The degree of displacement is the principal factor in determining treatment and prognosis. When the displacement is diagnosed early and treated effectively the prognosis is generally good. Coxarthrosis may appear as a subsequent outcome.

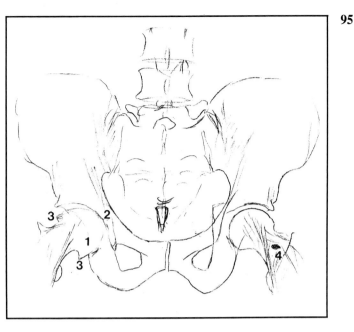

95

96 Osteopoikilosis

Multiple dense islets in the neck of the femur, the pubic rami, ilium and sacrum.

Osteopoikilosis is a rare hereditary disorder of bone characterised by multiple islets of dense bone, usually asymptomatic. In this patient a spondylolisthesis, causing his backache, was also diagnosed. Isolated islets of dense bone are often seen in the neck of the femur. Multiple dense areas should also make one consider the possibility of osteoblastic bone secondaries. In the case of metastases the margins of the dense areas are not sharply defined, unlike those of osteopoikilosis. Furthermore, osteopoikilosis should not be mistaken for tuberous sclerosis.

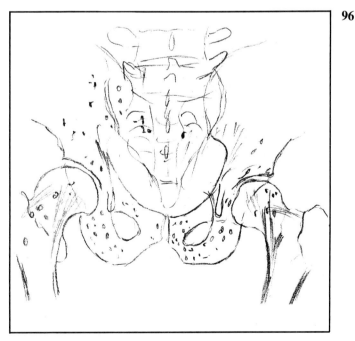

96

97

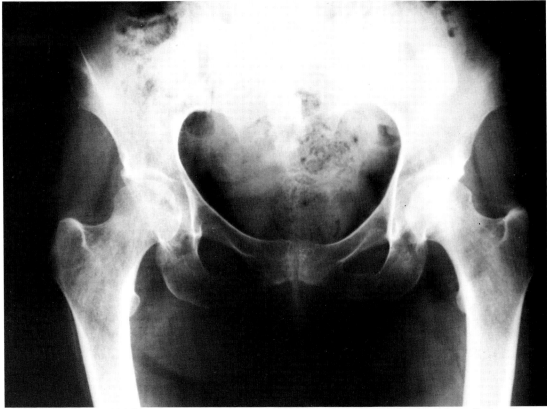

97 64 year-old housewife laid up for several months because of severe pain in the right leg. Right lower limb moist, cyanotic.

98

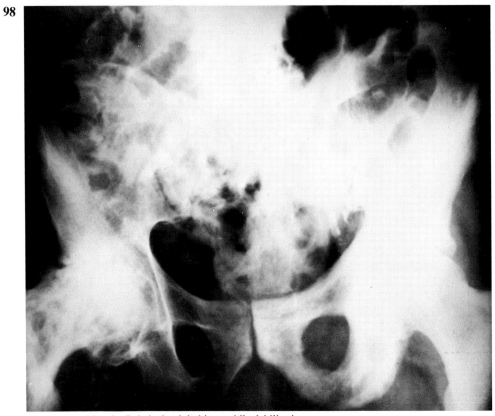

98 60 year-old male. Pain in the right hip, rapidly debilitating.

97 Algoneurodystrophy

Diffuse osteoporosis of the upper third of the right femur (1), and ilium (2). Joint space normal.

Algoneurodystrophy usually affects the upper limb (shoulder-hand syndrome) but may also occur in the lower limb. Algoneurodystrophy is in the majority of cases a complication of light trauma, as described by Südeck and Leriche. In addition to a very painful incapacity of the affected part (arm or leg) one observes the appearance of rapid and diffuse decalcification of bone and vasomotor disorders with trophic changes in the soft tissues (oedema, perspiration and cyanosis). The symptoms may persist for as long as two years and eventually disappear. The syndrome is usually based on a psycholabile personality.

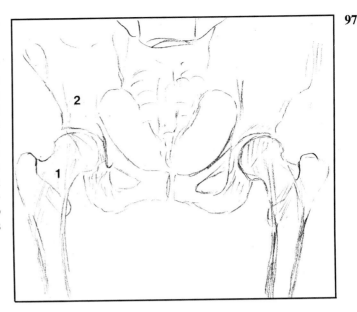

98 Paget's disease

Narrowed joint space of the right hip (1) with disorderly bone structure of the head and neck of the right femur (2), cyst formation (3), expansion of the neck of the femur with varus deformity (4), modified bone structure of the pubic rami with expansion (5), diffuse sclerosis (6), accentuated arcuate line (7), sclerosis and expansion of L4 (8), diffuse involvement of the sacrum (9).

Paget's disease or osteitis deformans is characterised by an excessive metaplastic process of bone which develops in a disorderly fashion and results in disorganisation of bone structure with a mixture of sclerosis and osteolysis. The disease may remain confined to one area but can also become dispersed to involve all bony tissue.

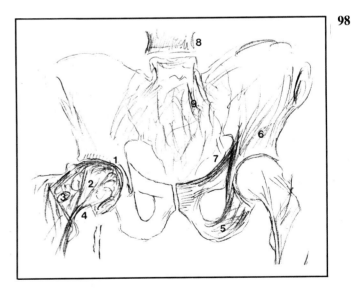

99

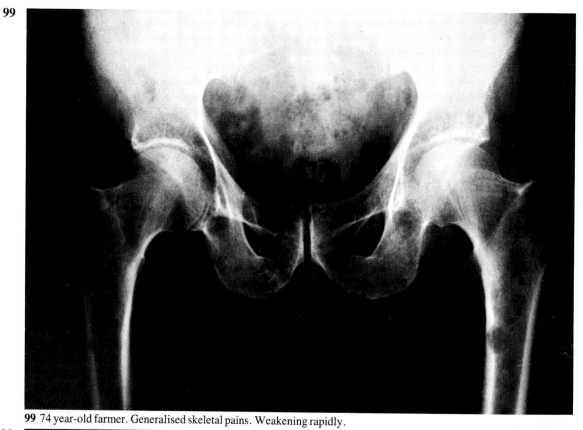

99 74 year-old farmer. Generalised skeletal pains. Weakening rapidly.

100

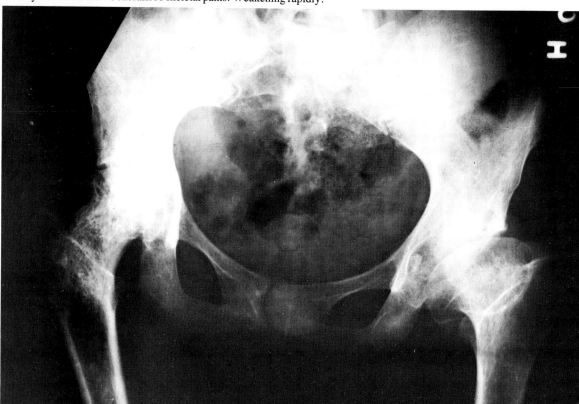

100 30 year-old housewife. Acute pain in the right thigh. Previously prolonged bout of pain in the left hip region. Splenectomy at the age of 9.

99 Multiple myelomatosis – Kahler's disease

estructive process in the shaft of the left femur
().

eneralised bone pain in the aged should suggest
ultiple myeloma. In this disease the radiologi-
al lesions are usually well demarcated; one sees
unched-out round rarefactions in the skull, pel-
is and long bones. On rare occasions, one may
nd generalised osteolysis accompanied by
ypercalcaemia.

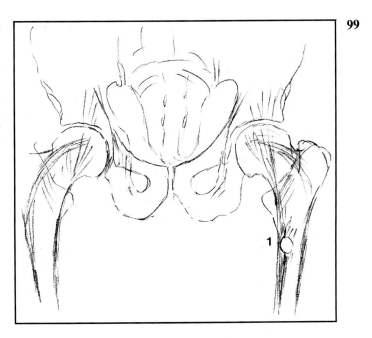

00 Gaucher's disease

lead of left femur flattened (1), neck of femur
hort (2), rounded translucencies and an area of
clerosis (crumbly appearance) in the head of the
ght femur (3), flattened upper surface with
mbankment of head of right femur (4).

aucher's disease is a very rare genetic disorder
haracterised by the presence of very large his-
ocytes filled with a lipoid, kerasin, in the haema-
poietic system – bone marrow, spleen, liver.

nvasion of Gaucher cells into bone causes
steolysis, swollen metaphyses and bony infarcts
ue to pressure on bloodvessels. The commonest
te for infarcts of bone to occur is the head of the
emur and of the humerus where one may see a
icture resembling aseptic necrosis.

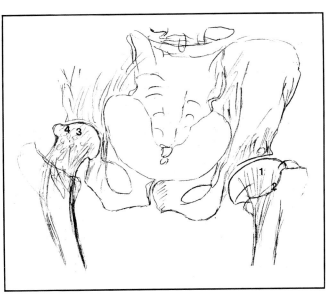

101

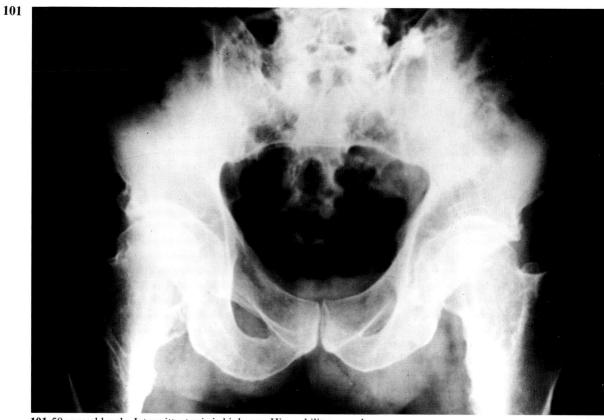

101 50 year-old male. Intermittent pain in his knees. Hip mobility normal.

102

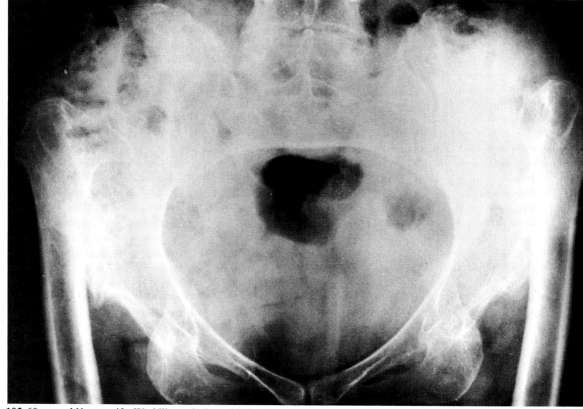

102 60 year-old housewife. Waddling gait since childhood.

101 Hereditary multiple exostosis – diaphyseal aclasia

Expansion and shortening of neck of femur (1), epiphysis of head of femur free from exostoses (2).

Hereditary multiple exostosis is an autosomal dominant bone abnormality marked by exostoses capped by cartilage occurring in the regions of growth cartilage. Affected patients sometimes have a small stature with shortening of the long bones.

Generally the exostoses do not cause complaints provided there is no pressure on a nerve or a vascular bundle. Sometimes the only accompaniment is an overlying bursitis. Malignant degeneration (chondrosarcoma) is rare.

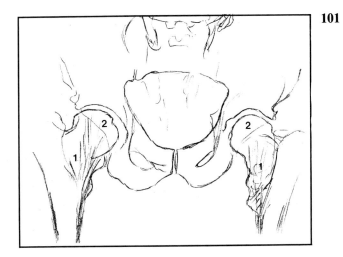

101

102 Congenital dislocation of the hip

Shallow acetabulum (1), complete dislocation of both hips (2), resorption of the head of the femur (3), with reconstruction of the neck of the femur (4), which forms a new fibrous joint with the ilium.

The abnormality, which exists from birth, is twice as common in breech than in vertex deliveries, occurs significantly more often in Italy and Scandinavia, presents 6-9 times more often in females than in males and heredity plays a role in 20 per cent of cases.

Thanks to a thorough examination of all newborn babies and because of treatment in abduction apparatus, the incidence of partial or complete dislocation of the hip has been radically reduced. Ortolani's sign (clicking) is diagnostic of dislocated hips in babies. With a thumb placed on the medial side of each knee the hips are moved into abduction while the other fingers press medially and upwards on the greater trochanters. Subluxation of the hip will produce a palpable and audible click.

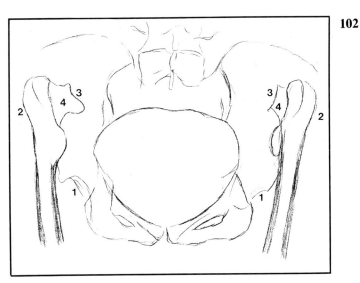

102

103

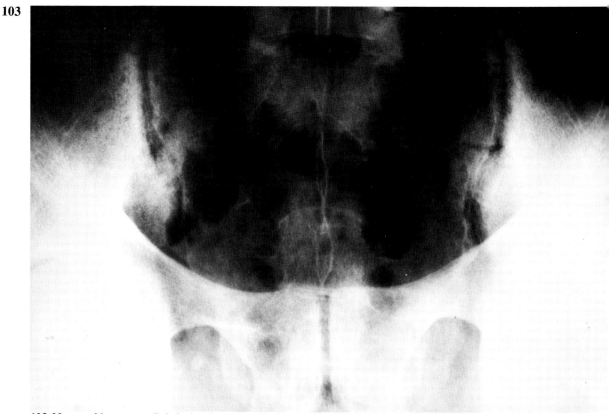

103 22 year-old carpenter. Pain in the gluteal regions, day and night, for 5 years. His sister is also being treated for backache.

104

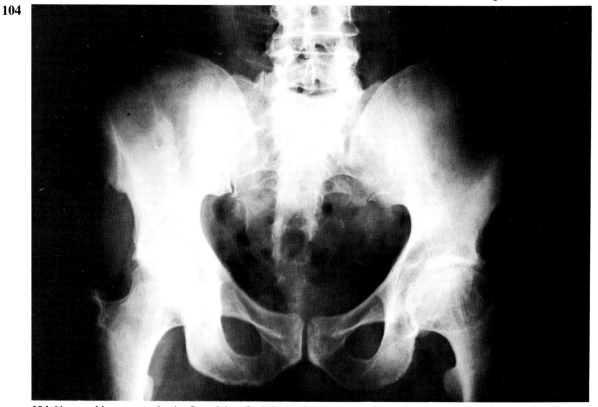

104 61 year-old garage mechanic. Complains of pain in the right lumbar region. At the age of 6 years he had a painful left hip which was immobilised in plaster.

03 Bilateral sacroiliac arthritis

lurred articular margins (1), widening of joint pace (2), erosion (3), bony bridge (4).

n encountering a bilateral sacroiliitis the first iagnosis considered is ankylosing spondylitis, echterew's disease. It should be noted however hat sacroiliac arthritis presents in a number of elated conditions which do not ankylose the ntire vertebral column: Reiter's disease, psoria- c spondylitis, juvenile rheumatoid arthritis, Crohn's disease and ulcerative colitis. In the latter wo conditions a completely asymptomatic sac- oiliitis sometimes exists. In all these conditions here is an increased frequency of occurrence of uman leucocyte antigen HLA B27.

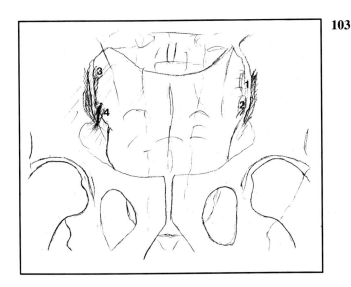

103

04 Coxa magna plana

lead of left femur wider and more rounded (1) nan that of the right, neck of femur wide and short 2).

his condition, coxa magna plana, is usually the esult of a treated or of a subclinical Legg- Perthes-Calvé disease which is an osteochondro- is (aseptic necrosis) of the head of the femur, in nost cases presenting in boys between the ages of and 8 years. It is sometimes caused by trauma. Following weight-bearing, the child complains of pain in the inguinal region, with moderate imitation of movement, especially abduction. The period of revascularisation and healing is bout three to five years, sometimes even longer.

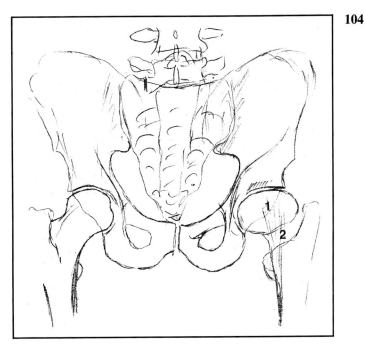

104

105

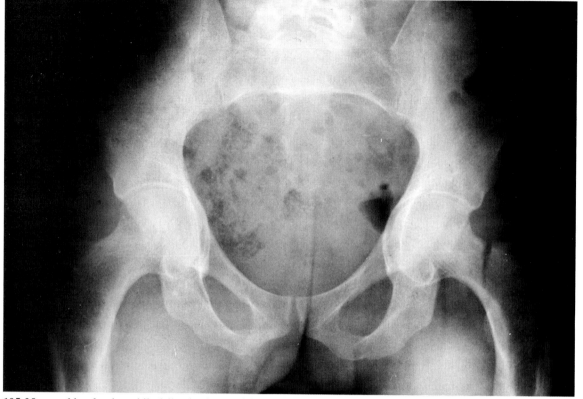

105 25 year-old male who, while delivering boxes of shoes, tripped on a small flight of stairs and then could not get up because intense pain in his left gluteal region.

106

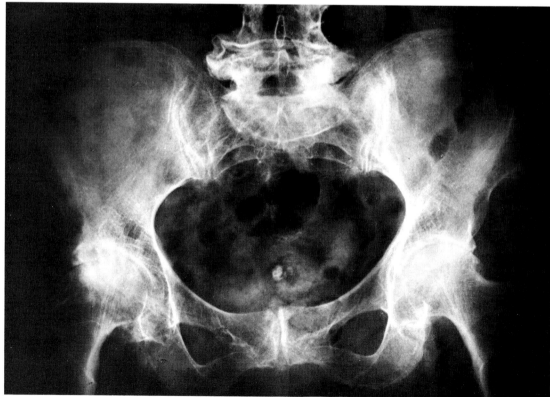

106 69 year-old woman with diabetes mellitus. Walks with difficulty because of increasing pain in the right hip. During the past few years her knees have swollen repeatedly.

05 Idiopathic protrusio acetabuli – fractured neck of femur with coxa vara

Fracture of neck of left femur (1), coxa vara with cervicodiaphyseal angle of 125 degrees (normal = 135 degrees) on the right (2), manifest bilateral protrusio acetabuli with excessively deep acetabulum, extending beyond the ischio-iliac line (3).

Idiopathic acetabular protrusion is an abnormality of growth during adolescence. As a result of altered biomechanical relations, a very debilitating coxarthrosis usually ensues. In this patient a fracture of the neck of the femur occurred, influenced by the abnormal biomechanics.

Secondary acetabular protrusion occurs in association with the following conditions: generalised osteoporosis, osteomalacia, osteogenesis imperfecta, Paget's disease, rheumatoid arthritis and cortisone therapy.

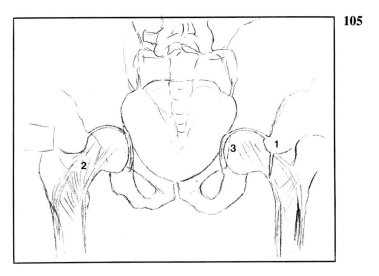

105

06 Coxarthrosis with chondrocalcinosis

Calcification of the fibrocartilaginous tissue of the pubic symphysis (1), bilateral narrowing of hip joint space (2), destruction of the right hip with signs of aseptic necrosis, depression (3), cyst formation (4), subchondral sclerosis (5), spondylosis with hypertrophic osteophytosis (6).

Chondrocalcinosis, Forestier type spondylosis with hypertrophic osteophytosis and aseptic necrosis of the femoral head are conditions that present more frequently in conjunction with diabetes mellitus than otherwise. The metabolic mechanism underlying these changes is not known at present.

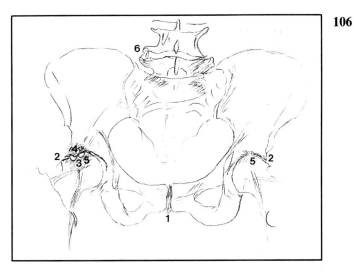

106

107

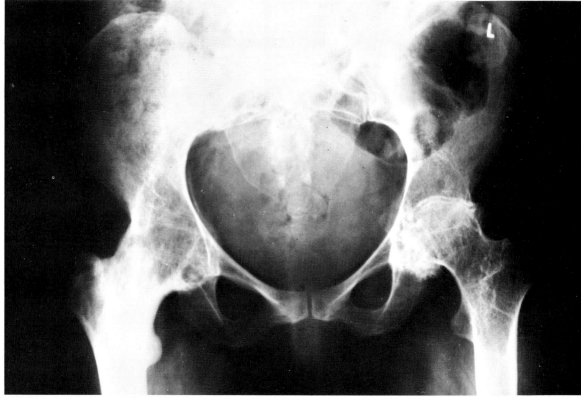

107 46 year-old spinster. Affected by polyarthritis since the age of 4. Has been in a wheelchair for 30 years and has not walked for years. She lives in a home for the aged.

108

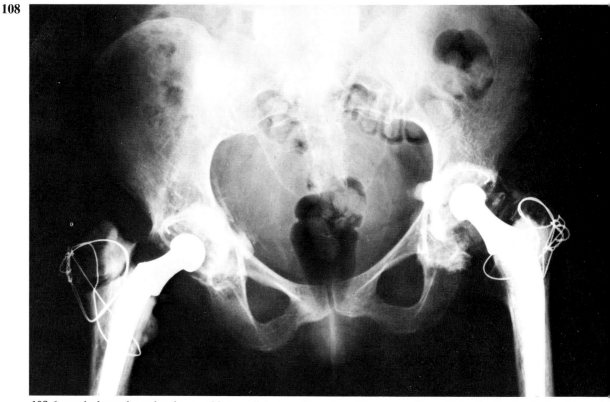

108 6 months later: the patient is now able to walk by herself, and now lives more often with her family than in the old people home.

07 Juvenile rheumatoid arthritis

ony ankylosis of right hip (1); on the left, coxitis ith overall diminution of joint space (2), teophytosis (3).

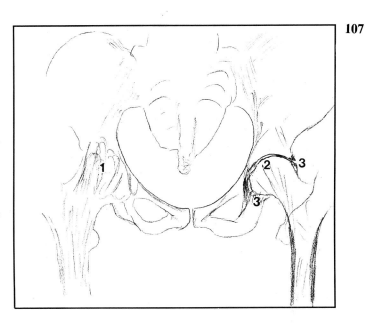

volvement of the hips occurs more commonly ith the juvenile than with the adult form of eumatoid arthritis. In juvenile rheumatoid thritis there is a greater tendency for ankylosis the joint to occur, hence the great importance of eping it mobile during the active phase and to oid forced positions. A coxitis is distinguished diologically from a coxarthrosis by the uniform minution of the joint space and by the atrophic, ecalcified appearance of the bone. In the case of oxarthrosis there is usually an uneven narrowing the joint space superolaterally and an associ- ed hypertrophic sclerosing reaction.

08 Total hip replacement

olyethylene acetabulum cups (1) and Vitalium moral head (2), transplantation of the greater ochanter (3).

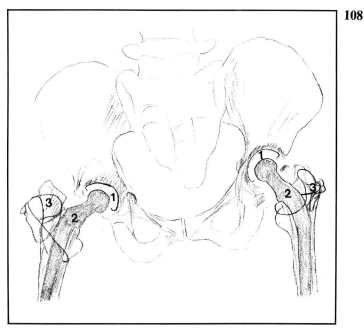

ver the last ten years the greatest step forward in constructive orthopaedics has been the intro- ction of total hip replacement for treating the ippling coxalgia due to coxitis or coxarthrosis. this manoeuvre the entire diseased joint is moved and replaced by a polyethylene socket d a metal (Vitalium) femoral head, anchored curely to the bone with a very solid adhesive bstance. The two parts of the hip prosthesis are different materials to prevent precocious detri- on. The postoperative recovery period is short nce the patient has regained a painless hip pable of total function.

he operation is tolerated well, even in the very d, and can be performed in very severe cases. In oung patients careful consideration of the in- cations for replacement is indicated due to lack knowledge regarding possible detrition and osening with time.

109

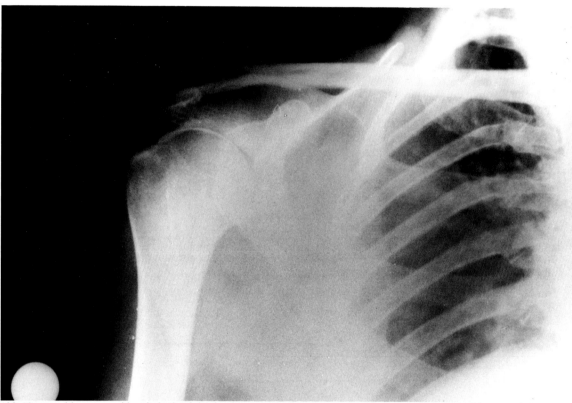

109 40 year-old woman with pain in the right shoulder at night for a few weeks. She cannot lie on this side or comb her hair, and dresses with difficulty.

110

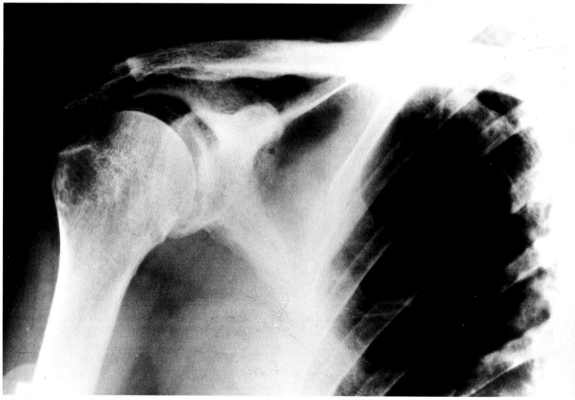

110 64 year-old spinster. Has had many years of treatment for recurring arthritis in various joints including knees, wrists and shoulders.

09 Calcifying supraspinatus tendinitis

alcification of supraspinatus tendon (1), scler-
sis of greater tubercle (2).

he radiological picture of a scapulohumeral
eriarthritis syndrome can vary widely. Typical
onormalities which do not however present in
very case are sclerosis of the greater tubercle,
alcification of the capsule, bursa or above all of
e supraspinatus tendon. Sometimes these signs
e seen in the contralateral asymptomatic
oulder.

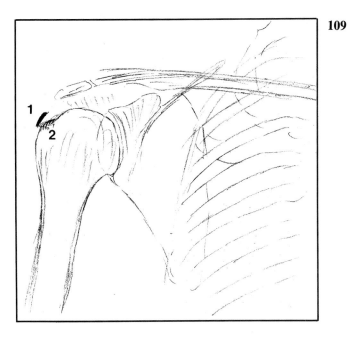

109

10 Chondrocalcinosis

ggshell calcification of the articular cartilage
), calcification of subacromial bursa (2), cal-
fication of the capsule (3).

hondrocalcinosis can be associated with a
vere arthritis due to calcium pyrophosphate
rystal synovitis. Usually the arthritis lasts for
ome weeks but may become chronic and produce
igns of articular degeneration like, in this case,
alcification of the bursa and capsule. With rup-
re of a calcified bursa one may witness the
evelopment of a very painful arthritis of the
houlder.

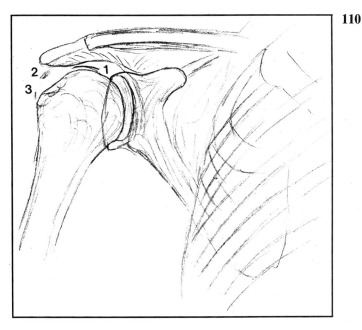

110

111

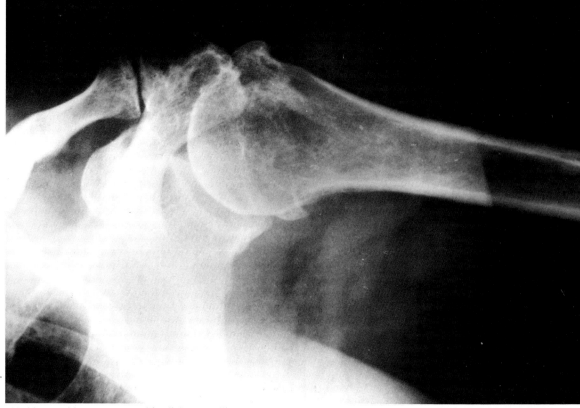

111 66 year-old woman, treated for diabetes mellitus. From time to time she has pain in the shoulder with limitation of movement

112

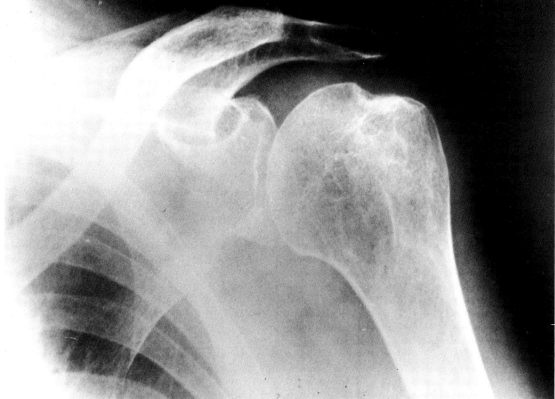

112 60 year-old female. Psoriatic polyarthritis.

111 Arthritis of the shoulder

Marginal osteophytosis (1), spongy subchondral sclerosis (2) with a few cysts (3), mild acromio-clavicular arthropathy (4).

Primary arthropathy of the shoulder is a rather rare condition. Generally the arthropathic manifestations are secondary to necrosis of the head of the humerus, chondromatosis, chronic arthritis and periarthritis. Patients suffering from diabetes mellitus show a strong tendency to develop osteophytic reactions and, with these, periarticular inflammation.

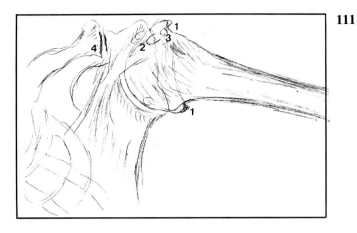

111

112 Psoriatic arthritis

Marginal erosion of the glenoid cavity (1) and of the anatomical neck of the humerus (2).

In the presence of an arthritis, erosions appear electively at the synovial reflexion where the membrane is attached to the bone. It is at these sites that the first radiological signs should be sought before there is any loss of cartilage. In the shoulder the loose nature of the capsule makes radiological demonstration of cartilage loss more difficult.

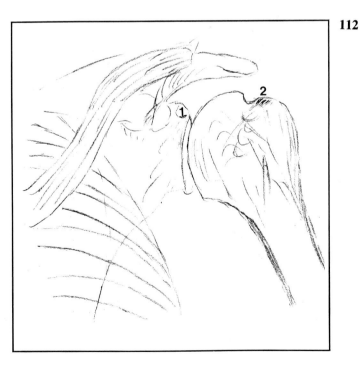

112

113

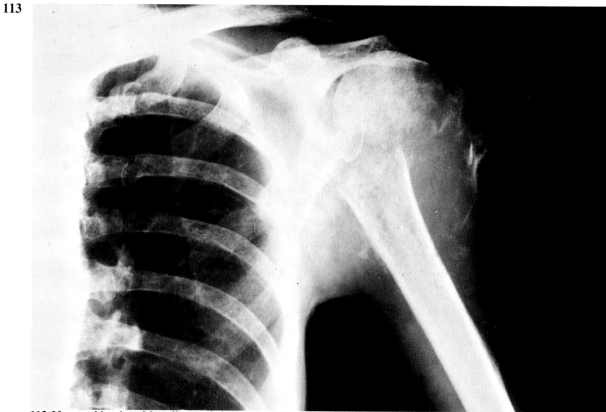

113 23 year-old patient. Mentally retarded. Pronounced swelling of the left shoulder and functional impairment of recent onset.

114

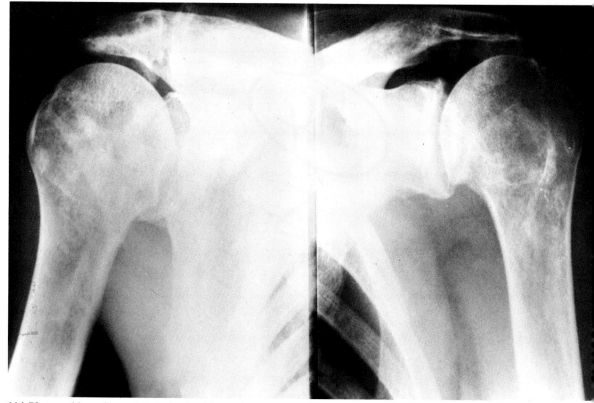

114 73 year-old pensioner. Pain in the shoulder and in the pelvic girdle day and night. Poor general condition. The clinical picture strongly suggests polymyalgia rheumatica.

113 Osteogenic sarcoma

Bone destruction with rupture of the cortex at the metaphysis of the humerus (1), bone formation within the tumour (2), periosteal spur (3), spontaneous fracture (4).

Osteogenic sarcoma is the commonest form of osteosarcoma and has a very poor prognosis even with radical amputation. The tumour usually occurs at the metaphysis of long bones and is characterised by osteoblastic activity within the tumour. This tumour presents most commonly in subjects between the ages of 10 and 20 years.

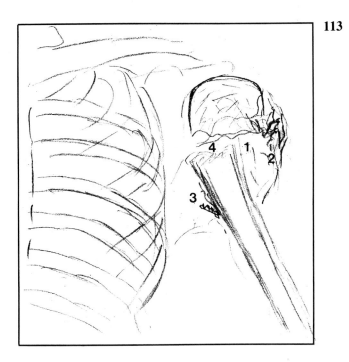

113

114 Osteoblastic secondaries from carcinoma of the prostate

Cloudy dense shadows (1) in the proximal one-third of the humerus bilaterally.

Shoulder pain presents frequently both in young and in old people. An exact diagnosis should always be sought for. In the differential diagnosis it is important always to exclude a malignancy with dissemination. The paraneoplastic myopathy strongly resembles rheumatic polymyalgia, a rheumatic disorder marked by an inflammatory girdle pain, an unsatisfactory general condition, a raised sedimentation rate and no signs of malignancy in old people, and also a positive response to corticosteroid therapy. In a certain number of cases, a temporal artery biopsy may show a giant cell arteritis.

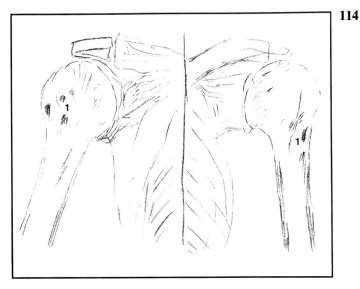

114

115

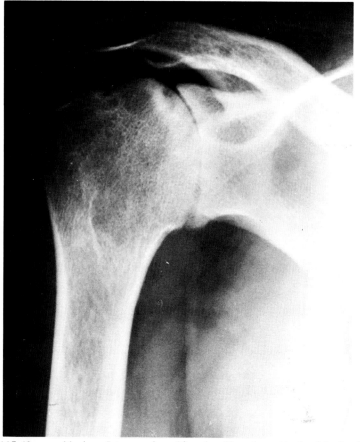

115 49 year-old miner. Intense pain and functional impairment in the right shoulder for 6 months. 20 years ago he suffered sciatica for several months. The patient is HLA B27 positive.

116

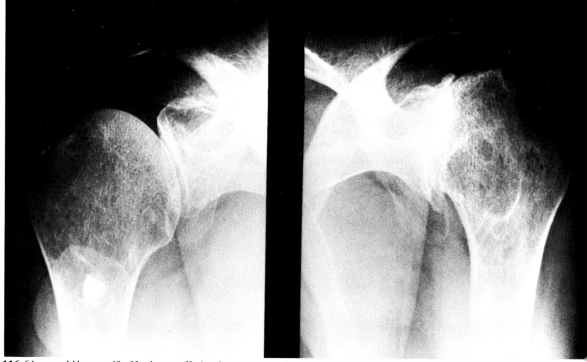

116 64 year-old housewife. Has been suffering from severe polyarthritis for 15 years.

15 Arthritis of the shoulder associated with spondylitis

Overall diminution of joint space (1) with erosion of upper and lower margins (2), subchondral sclerosis of both articular surfaces.

A monoarthritis of the hip or shoulder which persists for months should suggest the likelihood of an arthritis associated with one of the syndromes of pelvispondylitis like Bechterew's or Reiter's disease, psoriatic spondylitis or spondylitis accompanying a chronic intestinal inflammatory condition such as Crohn's disease or ulcerative colitis. In all these conditions there is often a history of iritis and the patients are likely to possess the HLA B27. In this particular case both sacroiliac joints were ankylosed and there was a ligamentous calcification, syndesmophyte, at T11-T12.

Likewise such a monoarthritis should always make one exclude the possibility of an infective cause such as tuberculosis. An examination of the synovial fluid and synovial biopsy are usually necessary in order to exclude the possibility of tuberculosis completely. In the early stages the radiological picture of articular tuberculosis is identical to that of a nonspecific arthritis: erosion, joint space diminution and periarticular osteoporosis.

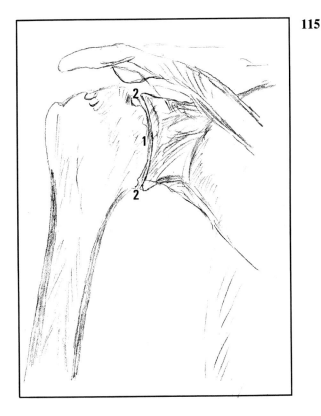

115

16 Rheumatoid arthritis

Slight narrowing of the right shoulder joint space (1), total obliteration of joint space (2) on the left with sclerosis of the articular margins (3), elevation of the head of the left humerus (4), erosions at the anatomical neck of the humerus (5).

Complete joint destruction with fibrous ankylosis due to rheumatoid arthritis, would produce less functional disability in the shoulder than in the hip. By reason of the mobility of the scapula, shoulder ankylosis is compensated to such an extent that most daily tasks can be carried out.

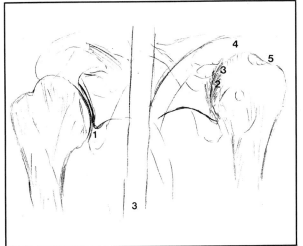

116

117

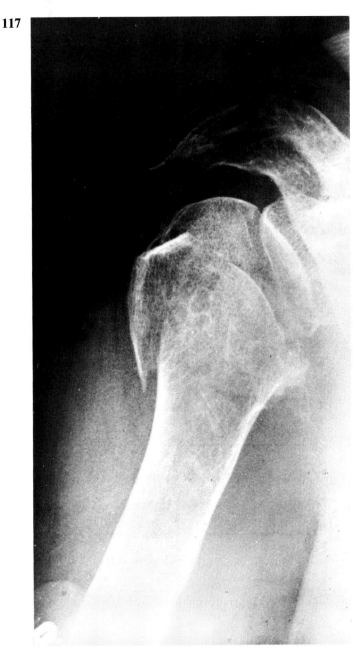

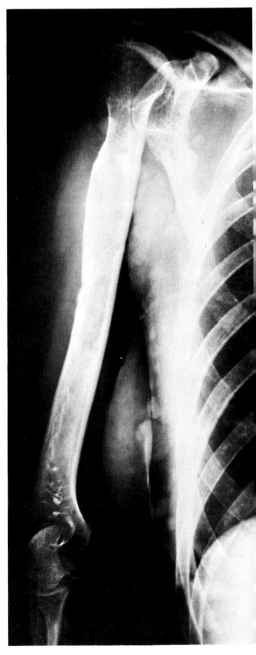

117 77 year-old peasant woman. Is being treated for an axial osteoporosis. She wakes up in the morning with pain in the right shoulder and limitation of movement.

118 52 year-old female. Pain in the right shoulder and severe limitation of movement. Multiple subcutaneous nodules. History of fractures of the humerus.

17 Pathological fracture of the neck of the humerus

Fracture of anatomical neck of humerus (1) and the greater tubercle (2) with abduction displacement of the shaft in relation to the elevated head.

Just as fracture of the neck of the femur with minimal trauma, fracture of the neck of the humerus likewise indicates a generalised osteoporosis.

Simple immobilisation of the shoulder and arm in plaster is sufficient treatment. Mobilising exercises should be instituted early in order to obtain a good functional result and to prevent a periarthritis or a shoulder-hand syndrome.

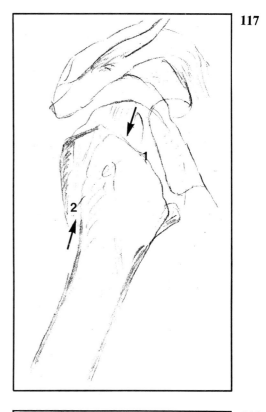

117

18 Von Recklinghausen's neurofibromatosis

Nodules in the soft tissues (1), old fracture of the neck of the humerus with displacement of the head (2), secondary capsulitis with elevation of the humeral head (3), frozen shoulder.

Von Recklinghausen's neurofibromatosis is a dominant autosomal hereditary abnormality characterised by the occurrence of café-au-lait stains of the skin and neurofibromas. Various bone abnormalities have been described in association with this disease: pseudoarthrosis of the tibia, cystic degenerations of bone, kyphoscoliosis, lacunar shadow of the skull and pressure erosion of ribs, vertebrae and skull. In very rare cases an osteomalacia with hypophosphoraemia and hyperphosphaturia has been reported.

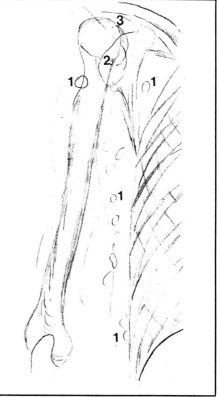

118

119

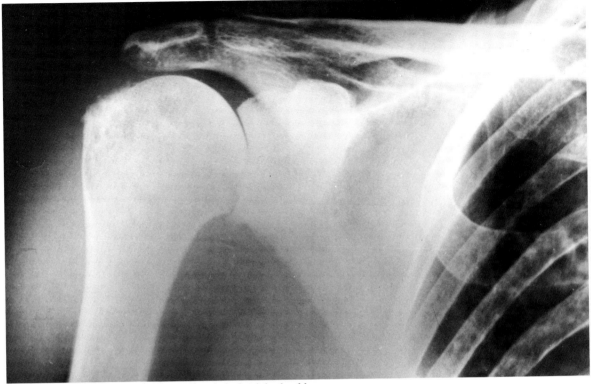

119 59 year-old tradeswoman. Treated for pain in the right shoulder.

120

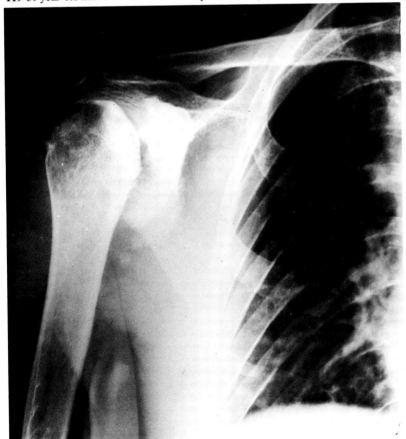

120 Two years later.

19 Neurogenic arthropathy with syringomyelia

oint space narrowing with blurred outlines and ıbchondral sclerosis (1), sclerosis with cystic ɛgenerations of the greater tubercle (2).

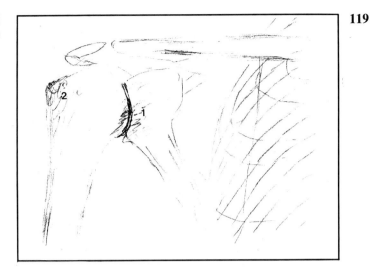

119

20

Destruction of the head of the humerus (1), regular outline and sclerosis of the glenoid avity (2), opacities in the soft tissues (3).

Because of its location in the cervical spinal cord nd altered sensation in the arm, syringomyelia vill cause a neurogenic arthropathy (Charcot's oint) in the upper limb. Radiologically eurogenic arthropathies present the following ommon characteristics: gross cartilage destruc- on with diminution of the joint space, marked ıarginal osteophytosis, osteosclerosis in areas of ressure, osteolysis of deeper structures, secon- ary osteochondromatosis. Because of repeated ıicrotrauma due to inertness of the joint, instabil- y of articular structures ensues and this promotes islocations.

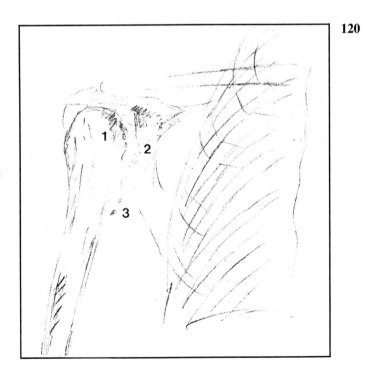

120

4: Knee and foot

nees and feet are subjected to a twofold requirement – support the weight of the body and to participate in the rocess of walking.

In addition to signs attributable to the causal malady, these joints also show the influence of mechanical factors, which adds to the form of the lesion and its radiological picture. Furthermore, distinct radiological differences may exist between a picture taken in the standing and one taken in the recumbent position.

The biomechanical functions of the knees and feet bring about anatomical effects which render the interpretation of radiographs difficult like superimposition of the patella, angulation of the ankle, flexed and extended position of the toes.

It is important to be aware of the position of the knees or of the feet in order to enable one to interpret radiographs of these joints accurately and thus avoid mistaken interpretations. As with other joints, comparison between left and right is necessary for recognising anatomical variations and for detecting early signs of disease.

Radiological examination reveals nothing, however, there are no structural alterations. Often radiological signs appear late. In the case of trauma, it is frequently necessary to take radiographs in different positions.

When visible lesions are detected on a radiograph, they are often pathognomonic, confirming a clinical diagnosis. Radiographs serve not only to validate a diagnosis but also to reveal the degree of damage and the stage of development of the disease.

121

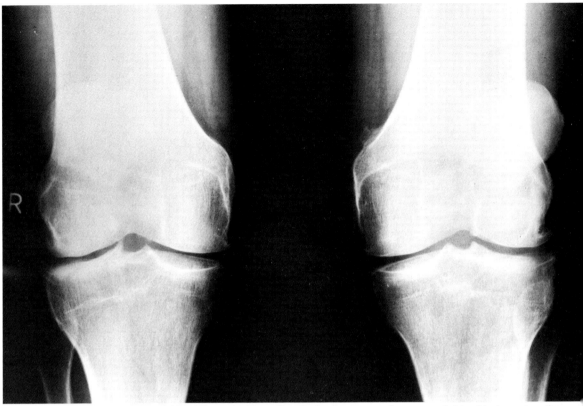

121 An obese 27 year-old pedlar weighing 98kg and 1.73m tall, suffering from a recurring monoarthritis of the knee since the age of 18.

122

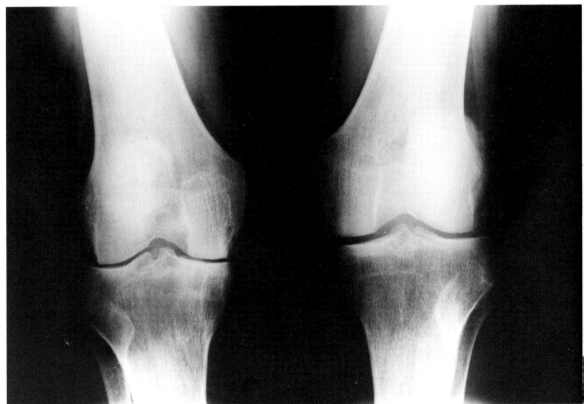

122 40 year-old female with painful swelling of the right knee for more than 6 months.

121 Gouty arthritis

Hypertrophic reaction of the bone with marginal osteophytosis (1), exostosis (2).

Gouty arthritis is a typical example of mono-arthritis which is crippling for a few days after which the pain subsides gradually.

Recurrent monoarthritis due to gout most commonly affects males between the ages of 20 and 40, and postmenopausal women. Tophi are late manifestations, presenting in untreated cases after about 10 years. There is no obvious correlation between the level of the blood uric acid and the frequency of acute attacks in gout. Many people have a moderately raised uricacidaemia without any symptoms. Gout cannot be diagnosed with any certainty unless microscopic examination of the synovial fluid reveals uric acid crystals phagocytosed by leucocytes.

Primary gout often occurs together with other metabolic disorders like hyperlipidaemia, diabetes mellitus and obesity.

The blood uric acid in this patient was 12.3mg per cent.

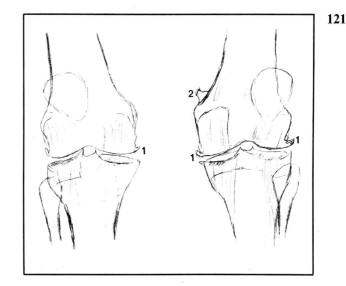

122 Rheumatoid arthritis

Uniform narrowing of the joint space (1), periarticular osteoporosis (2)

Monoarthritis often poses an important and intricate diagnostic problem. The problem is complicated because many rheumatic disorders can present chiefly with a monoarticular swelling. The problem is important because a wrong or delayed diagnosis can lead to serious and irreversible joint lesions, which can be averted by correct treatment as in septic or tuberculous arthritis.

The radiological signs of rheumatoid arthritis of the knee are not very specific. Apart from narrowing of the joint space which occurs late, one sees evidence of erosion in rare cases. The absence of osteophytosis and of sclerotic reaction would favour rheumatoid arthritis.

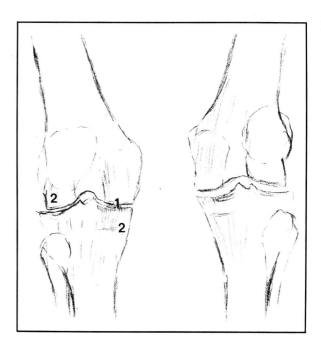

123

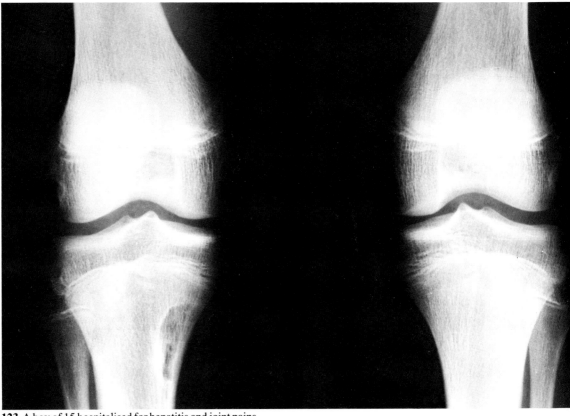

123 A boy of 15 hospitalised for hepatitis and joint pains.

124

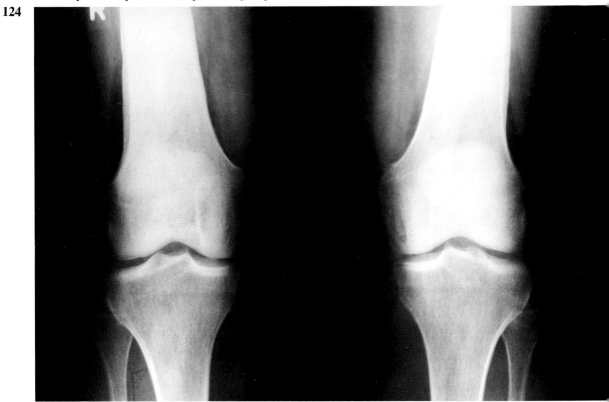

124 50 year-old male with nocturnal pain in the wrists, knees and ankles for about 20 months. He also has a chronic smoker's cou
and clubbed fingers.

123 Metaphyseal cortical defect – nonosteogenic fibroma

Intraosseous translucent area of the tibial diaphysis (1) with thinning of the overlying cortex (2) and a well-marked endosteal margin (3).

A metaphyseal cortical defect is an abnormality frequently encountered in children and adolescents and is often an incidental radiological discovery. The transparent area is, as a rule, situated in the metaphyseal region on the medial side of the tibia near the knee, or in the lower third of the femur. This is not a tumour. The translucent area contains yellowish brown fibrous tissue. On microscopic examination one sees connective tissue rich in collagen fibres, sprinkled with giant cells, but no new bone formation, hence the name nonosteogenic fibroma.

After a few years the cortical lacuna often disappears, sometimes leaving a sclerosed area. The picture is so characteristic that biopsy is unnecessary in most cases.

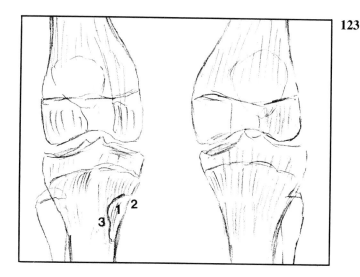

123

124 Hypertrophic pulmonary osteoarthropathy

Periosteal thickening, periostitis (arrow).

Arthralgia of the knees, ankles, elbows, wrists, lasting day and night, and periosteal reaction, can be the first manifestations of a malignancy hidden in the chest. In the case of a pulmonary carcinoma, the tumour may be small and difficult to diagnose. Hypertrophic osteoarthropathy can likewise occur with benign thoracic tumours and with secondaries in the lungs.

Periosteal reaction of the tibia may also be due to local irritation caused by phlebitis or subperiosteal haematomas.

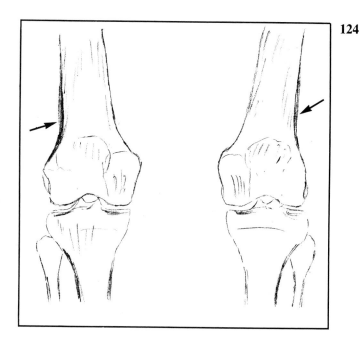

124

125

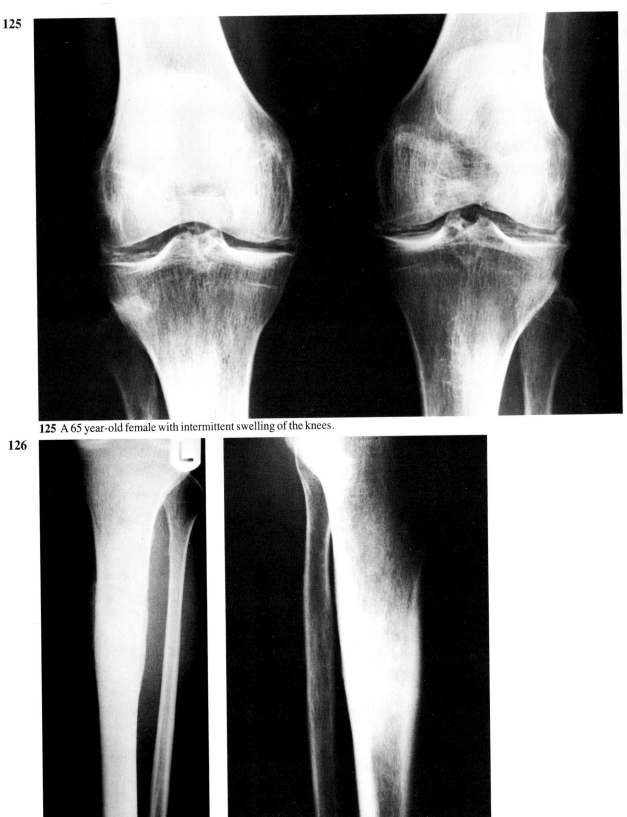

125 A 65 year-old female with intermittent swelling of the knees.

126

126 50 year-old lettuce grower. Complains of pain in the left knee and has a poor general condition. As a child he suffered periods of fever with pain in the legs.

125 Chondrocalcinosis – pseudogout

Meniscal calcifications (1), fragmented intracartilaginous calcification line throughout the joint (2).

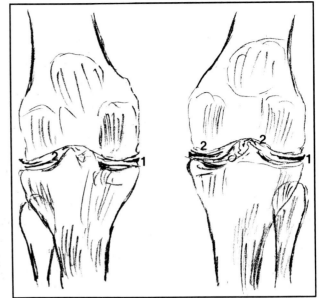

Chondrocalcinosis of the knees occurs frequently in old age. The calcifications are composed of calcium pyrophosphate dihydrate (CPPD) crystals, which can become liberated into the synovial fluid to give rise to a synovitis simulating an acute attack of gout (pseudogout). Pseudogout is only one of the various ways in which disease due to the precipitation of calcium pyrophosphate dihydrate crystals can manifest.
1. Pseudogout.
2. Pseudo-rheumatoid arthritis.
3. Pseudoosteoarthrosis.
4. Pseudoarthrosis with acute attacks.
5. Asymptomatic precipitation of CPPD crystals.
6. Pseudoneuropathic arthropathy.
The pseudo-rheumatoid arthritic form with chronic involvement of multiple joints is rare. Patients present most frequently with a combination of chondrocalcinosis and arthrosis. Whether it is in fact coincidental that chondrocalcinosis and arthrosis occur together is not clear.

Asymptomatic cases in which chondrocalcinosis is discovered by chance, occur in approximately 5 per cent of the older population. In these cases one should always look for an associated endocrine abnormality.

Finally one has to point out that destructive lesions of joints such as occur in neuropathic arthropathies can present in chondrocalcinosis.

126 Osteomyelitis

Periosteal reaction (1), osteosclerosis of upper third of tibial shaft (2).

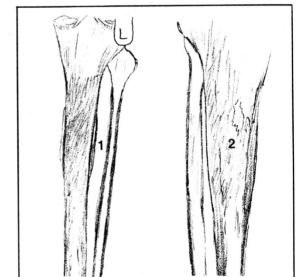

Osteomyelitis is often located in the metaphysis or metaphyseal transition zone, commonly around the knee. The disease occurs most frequently during adolescence and the majority of cases are caused by a bloodborne staphylococcal infection.

After spontaneous remission or successful antibiotic treatment, a recurrence of the disease may present years later, as in this case. At the onset of an acute attack radiography reveals no abnormality. In untreated cases a metaphyseal translucent area and periosteal reaction can be seen after a few weeks. When the osteitis becomes chronic, one sees the appearance of marked bone hypertrophy with periosteal reaction, irregular densities and radiotranslucent areas containing sequestra.

A centrally situated abscess of the tibial metaphysis, showing rounded cavities with small sequestra and walled in by an osteosclerotic area, is called a Brodie's abscess and must be evacuated. Sometimes osteomyelitis presents the picture of a focus of sclerosing osteitis without sequestrum formation.

127

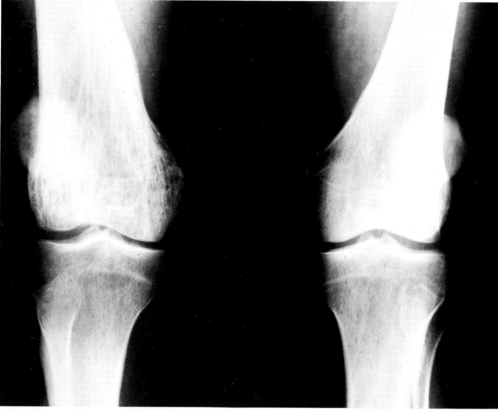

127 A 58 year-old baker with a painful right knee and progressive deformity of the lower limbs.

128

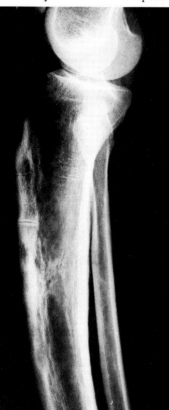

128 A 60 year-old civil servant complains of discomfort in his right leg which is becoming crooked and feels warm.

127 128 Paget's disease

127

Coarsegrained bone structure (1) with translucent areas and widening of the femoral metaphysis (2).

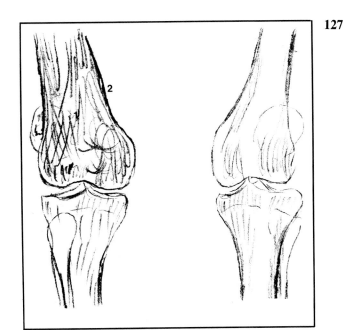

128

Hypertrophy and increased anterior curvature of the tibia (1), fibrillar and disorganised appearance of the bone trabeculae (2), fissure fractures anteriorly (3), lower third of tibia normal with V-shaped demarcation (4).

The bony abnormalities of Paget's disease can give rise to joint complaints. Bending of the femur produces a genu varum with abnormal weight distribution and ensuing secondary arthrosis. The curvature can also lead to fractures caused by minimal trauma. The fractures are usually transverse with smooth surfaces; callus formation is good. Radiography reveals incomplete fissures along the convex border. These fissures are usually painless.

Pagetoid bone changes are accompanied by a markedly increased blood demand with multiplication and dilatation of the small vessels. This produces an increase in local skin temperature, for example over the tibia, and may lead to cardiac decompensation if the pagetoid areas become widespread.

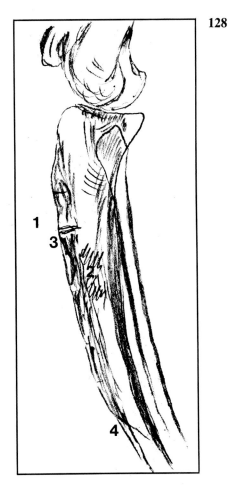

129

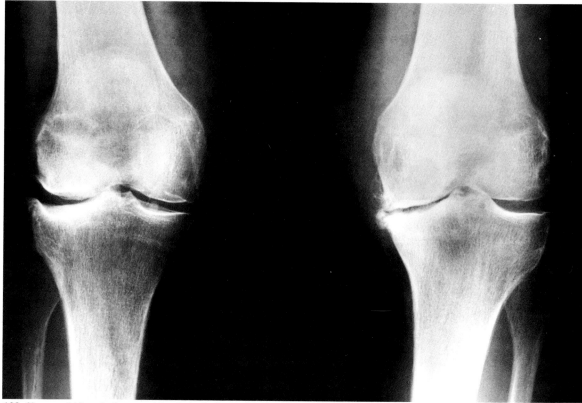

129 60 year-old female farmer with pain in the knees for 10 years, more in the right than in the left, especially on walking. Pictur taken in the recumbent position.

130

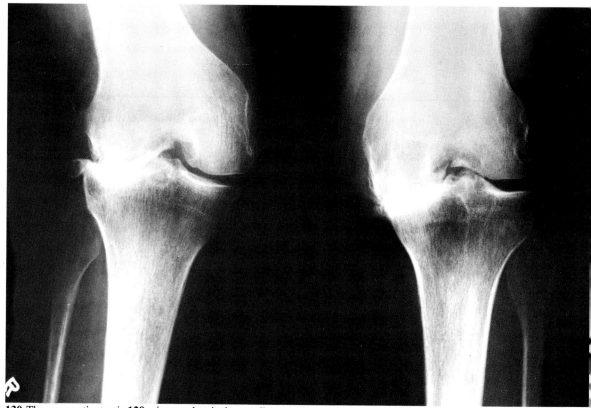

130 The same patient as in **129**, picture taken in the standing position.

129-130 Gonarthrosis

129

Uneven joint space narrowing (1), osteosclerosis and osteophytic reactions (2), depression of tibial plateau (3), accentuation of intercondylar tubercles (4), genu varum on the left (5), genu valgum on the right (6).

Arthrosis of the knee is usually bilateral and can be primary or secondary. The commonest causes of a secondary arthrosis are genu varum, genu valgum, and recurrent disclocation or subluxation of the patella.

The earliest signs of primary gonarthrosis present after the age of 40 and mostly after 50. Most patients are females. They are frequently obese and have obvious varicose veins of the legs. The main complaint is pain brought on by walking, subsiding with rest. Climbing up and down stairs is particularly painful.

The first radiographic signs are accentuation of the intercondylar tubercles, osteophytosis of the upper and lower margins of the patella and osteophytosis of tibial and femoral condyles, front and back, to be seen on a lateral view. Later marked narrowing of the joint space, osteophytosis of the lateral margins and subchondral sclerosis with cyst formation will become evident.

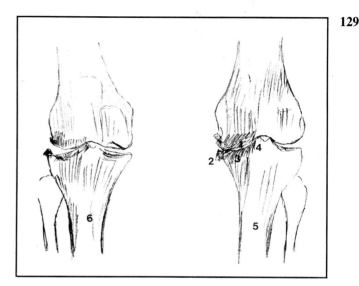

129

130

Note the importance of weight bearing to gauge the biomechanical position and the thickness of the cartilage.

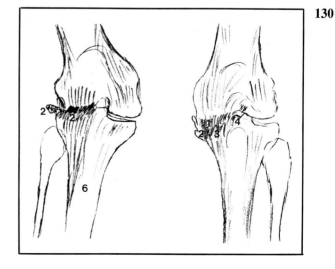

130

131

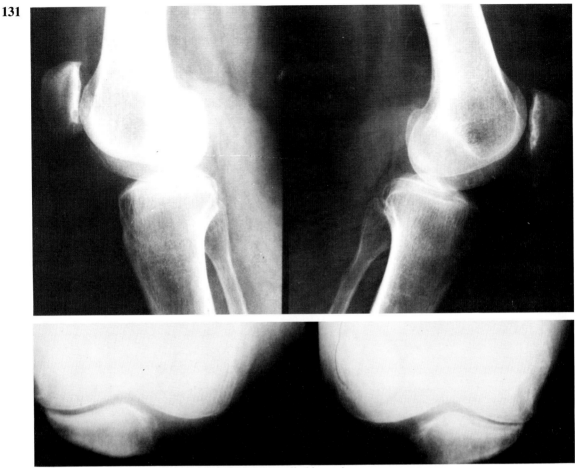

131 A 56 year-old seamstress with pain in the knees on climbing stairs.

132

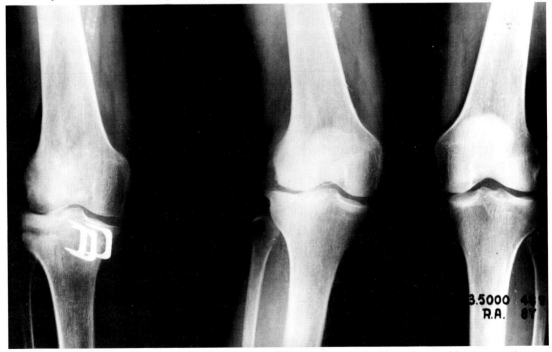

132 48 year-old female with polyarthritis since the age of 8, wrongly treated with corticosteroids. A corrective operation was performed on the right knee for pain on weight bearing and instability.

31 Patellofemoral dysplasia and gonarthrosis

. Lateral view: posterosuperior osteophytosis
1), subchondral cystic areas (2).

. Axial view : joint space diminution laterally
1), osteophytosis (2), dysplasia of the patellar
urface of the femur (3). Normally the angle made
y the two slopes of the patellar surface is at most
40 degrees and the lateral condyle projects for-
ard .5cm more than the medial.

atellofemoral dysplasia can give rise to recur-
ent dislocation and subluxation of the patella
vith ensuing degeneration of the cartilage (chon-
romalacia). With chondromalacia, the patient
xperiences pain on descending a staircase, on
ercussing the patella and on pressing the patella
iterally. In time radiological signs of gonarthro-
is appear. Special axial radiographs of the patella
re needed to demonstrate patellofemoral dyspla-
ia. In case of serious dysplasia, surgical correc-
on with transposition of the tibial tuberosity can
revent or improve secondary arthrosis. In
ome patients good quadriceps exercises may
uffice to correct the position of the patella in
elation to the femur.

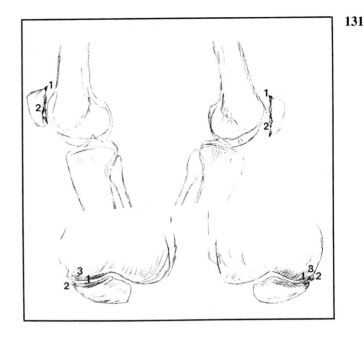

32 Rheumatoid arthritis – secondary arthrosis

Jneven diminution of joint space (1), depression
f the tibial plateau (2), genu valgum (3),
steophytosis (4), marginal erosions (5), varus
romoting osteotomy (6).

Persistent pain in the knee with disability can set
n as a result of laxity of the joint through loss of
artilage, stretching of the capsule and depression
f a supporting surface. This anomaly, with poor
natomical posture, is best treated surgically. The
natomical disruption cannot be corrected by the
njection of cortisone or with painkilling drugs,
vhich may even be dangerous. Anatomical re-
onstruction is possible by elevating one of the
upporting surfaces, introducing an elevating
rosthesis or by total knee replacement.

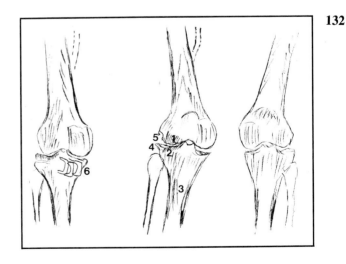

133

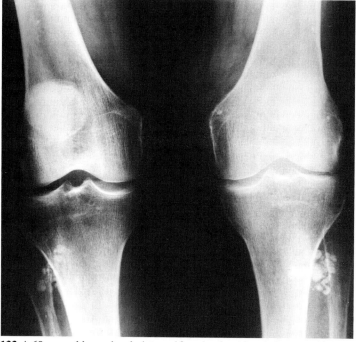

133 A 60 year-old nun, headmistress of a school, with pain in several joints for many years. She is being treated for rheumato arthritis.

134

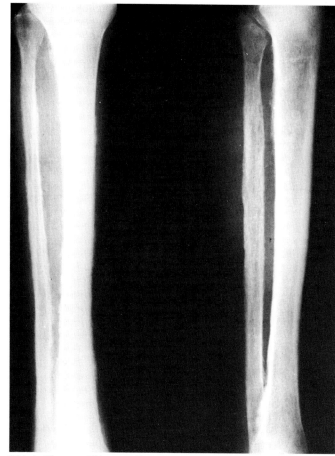

134 A 55 year-old housewife with a 12 year history of polycythaemia vera, now presents with anaemia, splenomegaly ar thrombocytopaenia.

33 Bursitis calcarea

Infrapatellar and pretuberal calcifications (1), uniform joint space narrowing (2) through rheumatoid arthritis.

By repeatedly subjecting a particular area to the pressure of weight bearing, chronic reactive bursitis may be caused in the bursae of the area with ensuing calcification. This anomaly was formerly often seen in persons who kneel a lot like clergymen (parson's knee), charwomen who polish floors on their knees (housemaid's knee) and miners.

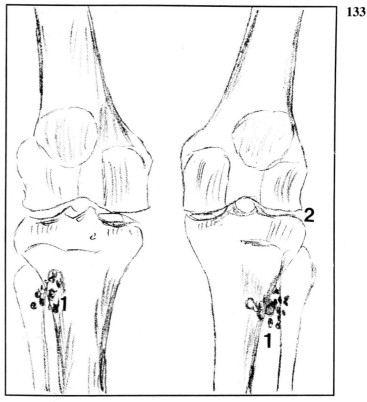

133

34 Myelofibrosis – periostitis

Diffuse sclerosis (1), periostitis (2), no well marked difference between cortex and medulla.

The periostitis of long bones in myelofibrosis is caused by subperiosteal bleeding with thrombocytopaenia. With vitamin C deficiency in children (scurvy) one finds similar widespread periosteal reactions to subperiosteal bleeding.

The radiological signs of myelofibrosis depend on the stage of the disease. At first one sees either diffuse osteoporosis in the medullary region or radiotranslucent areas in the bone marrow which will later sclerose. As the bone forming reaction progresses the density of the bone increases and may invade all the cancellous bone until the distinction between cortex and medullary cavity is obliterated.

The diagnosis of myelofibrosis can eventually only be confirmed by marrow biopsy.

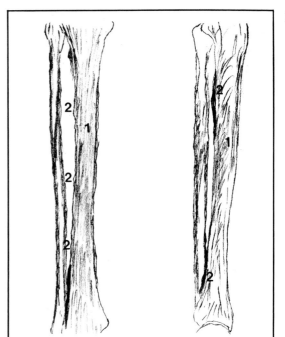

134

135

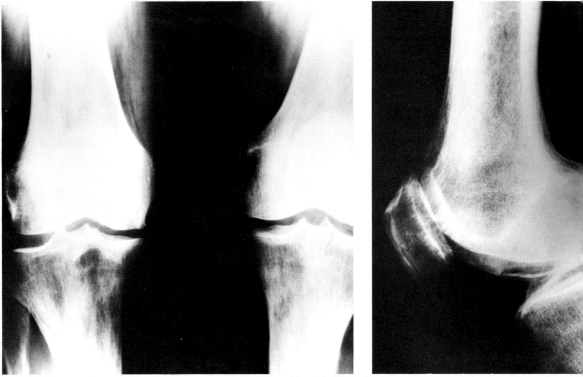

135 A church missionary of 73 with severe pain and disability of the right knee which came on suddenly in Hong Kong. Thereafter the right knee has locked three times.

136

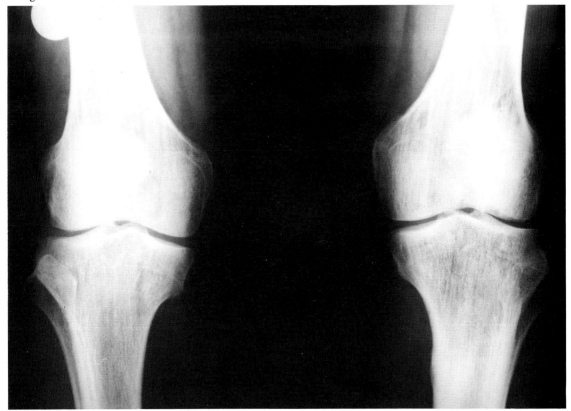

136 43 year-old female with multiple congenital abnormalities: small stature, asymmetry of the face, syndactyly, super-numerary toes, moderate deafness, dystrophic nails and atrophic skin with pigmentation and telangiectasis. She complains of pain in the left knee on weight bearing.

135 Aseptic necrosis – osteochondritis dissecans

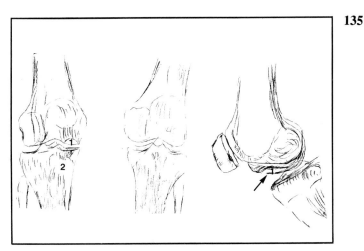

Semilunar translucency (1), medial condyle of right femur, mottled translucent area below medial condyle of tibia (2).

One should consider osteonecrosis of the medial femoral condyle in elderly people who present with a monoarticular knee complaint after minimal trauma. Osteonecrosis of the femoral condyle in the aged is distinguished by its position from osteochondritis dissecans which occurs in young people.

In osteonecrosis the lesion is situated towards the middle of the condyle, in the weight bearing area while in juvenile osteochondritis the anomaly occurs nearer the intercondylar notch.

The onset is usually associated with mild trauma. Osteonecrosis occurs most frequently in women, especially after 60. The knee is as a rule moderately swollen, with effusion. In the later stages locking may occur if a fragment of bone becomes detached. During the first weeks no radiographic lesion is evident. Thereafter a typical semilunar shadow appears as described above. Bone scintography reveals a localised concentration of the isotope.

136 Osteopathia striata

Fine, parallel lines (1) of dense bone running from epiphysis to metaphysis into the diaphysis. On the medial side of the left tibia the outcome of stress fracture (2) can be seen.

Osteopathia striata, also sometimes called Voorhoeve's disease, is a rare, asymptomatic abnormality usually discovered on radiological investigation. The striations consist of fine lines issuing from the metaphysis and extending into the epiphysis and diaphysis. The knee region is most frequently affected and the condition is bilateral.

The etiology is unknown. There is some evidence that this is a dominant hereditary condition. Osteopathia striata is often associated with other skeletal and skin abnormalities. Thus the concurrence with osteopoikilosis and focal dermal hyperplasia (Golz syndrome) is noted, as in this patient. Osteopathia striata is therefore an expression of ectomesodermal dysplasia.

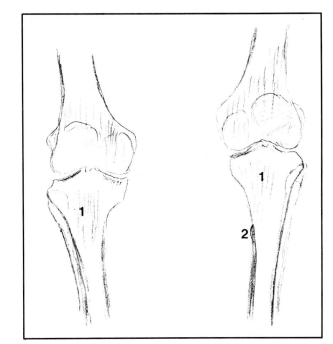

137

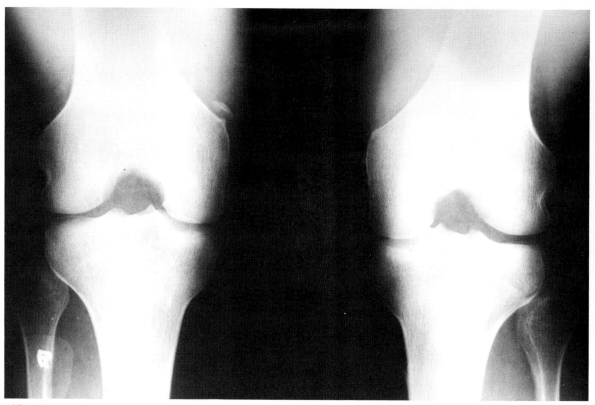

137 A 30 year-old garage mechanic; amateur water skier. Past history of recurrent dislocation of the shoulder, dislocation of the hip, and now a torsion injury of the right knee.

138

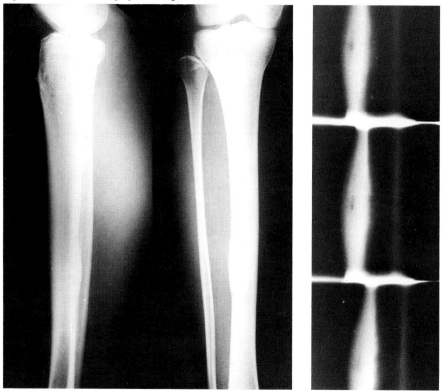

138 22 year-old psychology student; ballet dancing as a hobby, complains of pain in the right leg about the middle of the tibia, for 6 months. The pain is not aggravated by movement. She is particularly troubled at night and while sitting. The pain is eased by aspirin.

137 Pellegrini Stieda disease – post traumatic ossification

Paracondylar calcification (1).

Pellegrini Stieda's disease falls within the framework of post traumatic paraarticular ossifications and presents, as radiological characteristic, a calcification near the medial femoral condyle. This calcification establishes itself gradually after strain of the tibial collateral ligament. The lesion often remains painless.

This condylar radiograph differs from the usual anteroposterior view by its special angle of incidence from behind with the knees slightly flexed and the patient in the prone position. The condylar view reveals the back of the condyles better, also giving a better picture of the intercondylar area with the intercondylar eminence of the tibia. The usual anteroposterior view exposes particularly the weight bearing areas and thus the articular surfaces of the condyles where the lesions of osteochondritis dissecans arthropathy and arthritis are situated.

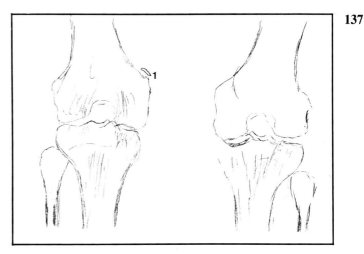

137

138 Osteoid osteoma

Thickening of the tibial cortex laterally and posteriorly (1), tomographic examination reveals central cystic areas (2).

Osteoid osteoma is a benign tumour of connective tissue with bone forming osteoblasts. The tumour itself is small, 0-2cm in diameter, but evokes bone proliferation in its vicinity especially in the cortex of long bones. Osteoid osteoma occurs most frequently in adolescents and young adults and affects particularly the lower limbs. There is a definite pain which causes trouble mostly at night, and is eased by aspirin.

Radiologically one sees a thickening of the bone with a central translucent area where the tumour is situated. Sometimes there is a central calcification, or nidus, within the translucent zone. When the tumour occurs in cancellous bone there is little bone thickening. In cortical bone the central translucent area may not be visible because of bone density and can only be demonstrated on tomography.

Treatment consists of curettage or excision depending on the site. Spontaneous cure may occur after 2-4 years. Differential diagnosis includes stress fracture and osteomyelitis.

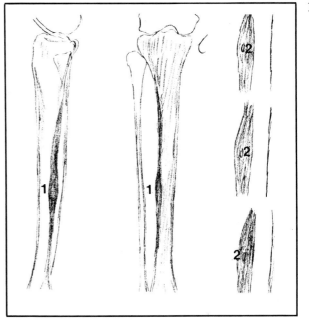

138

139

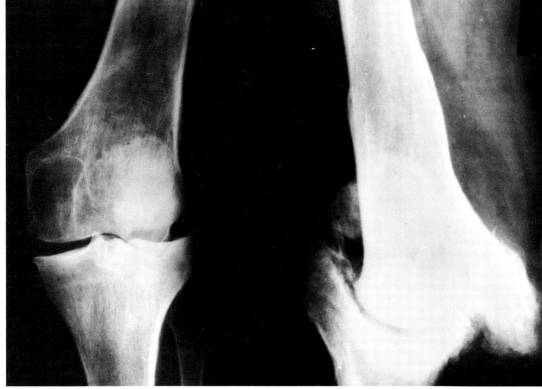

139 A 68 year-old innkeeper with instability of the right knee and bilateral flat feet. Despite 4 years increasing valgus deformity she can still walk 5km and even dances in her inn from time to time.

140

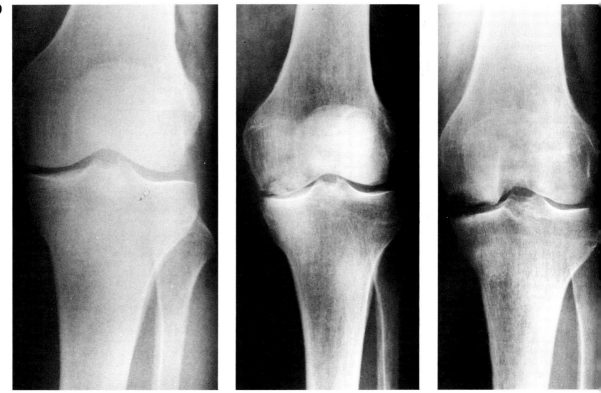

140 80 year-old lady who developed a sudden pain in the left knee after stumbling. Owing to persistent trouble an Xray picture (left) was taken and intraarticular cortisone was injected repeatedly. 8 weeks later increase of pain and swelling plus a raised temperature. The second picture was taken. 10 weeks later after intensive antibiotic therapy the third picture was taken.

139 Neuropathic arthropathy

Development of a tabes dorsalis type neuropathic joint over a period of 4 years.

A. Uneven joint space diminution laterally with valgus deformity (1), marginal osteophytosis (2), subchondral sclerosis (3).
B. Grave joint destruction with medial displacement (1), osteocartilaginous loose bodies (2), resorption of femoral condyles (3), periosteal reaction (4).
Previously tabes was the prime cause of neuropathic arthropathy. Even now it presents occasionally.

Tabetic neuroarthropathy affects the lower limbs exclusively, in particular the feet, attacking the midtarsal joint and sometimes accompanied by a perforating ulcer of the sole. The ankle, knee and hip are also affected. Less frequently the lumbar spine is involved.

Neuroarthropathy of the lower limbs, especially the feet, is now usually the result of a diabetic neuritis. In leprosy one may see similar neuropathic arthropathies of the feet and ankles.

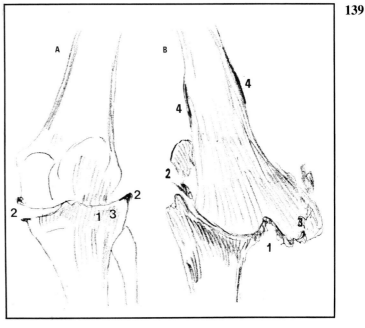
139

140 Septic arthritis – aseptic necrosis

Radiograph I: normal knee; Radiograph II: biconcave sequestrum (1) surrounded by a radiotranslucent zone (2); Radiograph III: diminution of the joint space (1), marginal erosion (2), empty niche (3).

Iatrogenic septic arthritis is nowadays commoner than that caused by blood dissemination. Staphylococcus aureus is the most frequent causal organism. Septic arthritis is most often based on an existing joint disease such as rheumatoid arthritis, gout and lupus. Every intraarticular injection or puncture carries the risk of introducing a bacterial infection, and increasingly so as more frequent joint aspiration is practised and cortisone injected.

One should suspect a septic arthritis in every case of painful monoarthritis where there is an accompanying deterioration of the general condition. Swift diagnosis and treatment are of the greatest importance since loss of time results in serious and irreversible destruction of cartilage. For the sake of diagnosis aspiration is indicated in order to identify the causal agent.

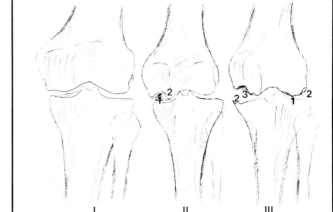
140

141

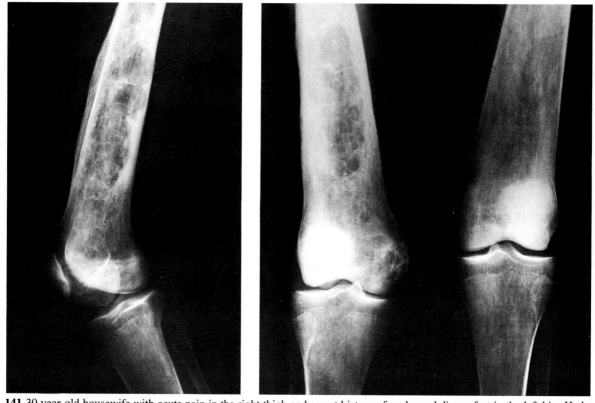

141 30 year-old housewife with acute pain in the right thigh and a past history of prolonged discomfort in the left hip. Had a splenectomy when 9 years old.

142

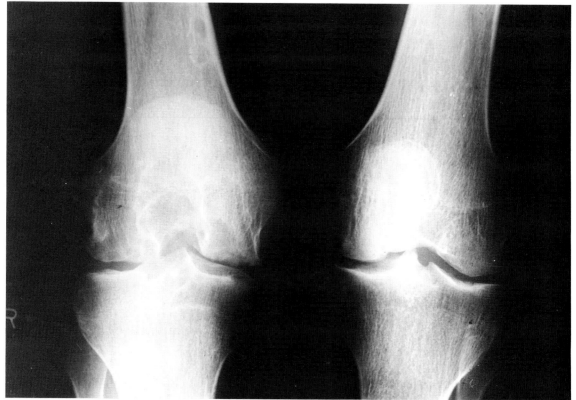

142 21 year-old student of dentistry who has been treated for intra-articular bleeding since the age of 9. For the last few months, weekly bleeding into the right knee.

141 Gaucher's disease

Hypertrophy of the lower third of the femoral shaft (1), endosteal erosions (2), geodes (3), periosteal reaction (4).

The bony lesions of Gaucher's disease are due to the invasion of the bone marrow by Gaucher's cells. Bony abnormalities are often latent but on the other hand may give rise to bone pain and spontaneous fractures. The lesions affect tubular bones, which become osteoporotic with oval translucencies and endosteal erosions. The metaphyseal area acquires a blown up appearance. Expansion of the lower femoral shaft produces an outline resembling an Erlenmeyer flask.

Aseptic necrosis ascribed to compression and obstruction of bloodvessels occurs frequently.

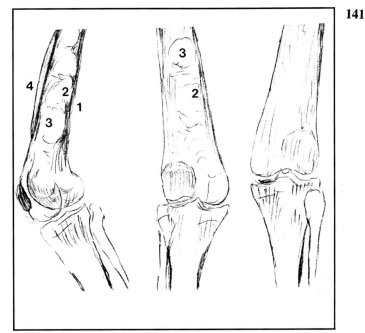

141

142 Arthropathy with haemophilia

Erosions (1), subchondral cystic translucencies and appearance of cavitation (2), joint space diminution (3), widening of intercondylar notch (4), widening of distal femoral epiphysis (5), intraosseous cystic translucencies (6).

Bleeding into joints is a complication which often occurs in haemophyliacs following minimal trauma. These synovial haemorrhages occur principally in the knees and are usually recurrent. Bleeding into a joint cavity generates a chronic inflammatory reaction with haemosiderosis in the synovial tissues. This inflammation leads to loss of cartilage, subchondral cystic degeneration and growth disorders in the bone and because of these abnormalities the term haemarthrosis has come into use.

In Willebrand's angiohaemophilia and also with anticoagulant therapy, haemarthrosis is encountered much less commonly.

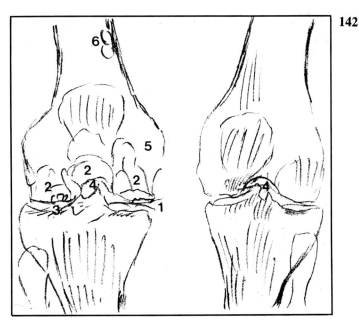

142

143

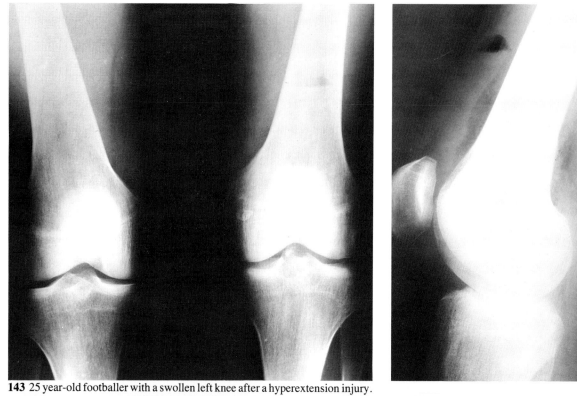

143 25 year-old footballer with a swollen left knee after a hyperextension injury.

144

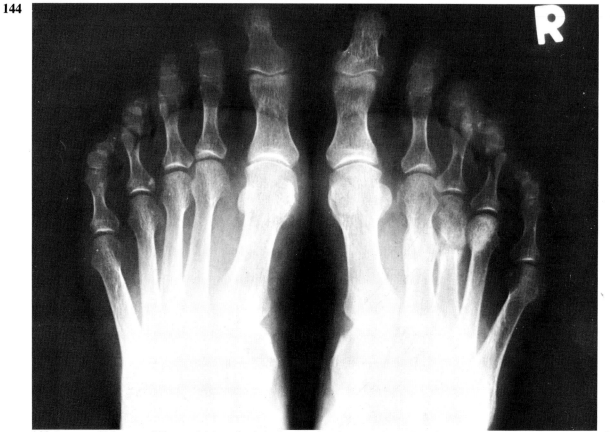

144 A seasonal labourer of 60 complaining of pain in the right foot for several months. 10 years ago had a partial gastrectomy for ulcer.

143 Intraarticular fracture

Loose fragment of medial intercondylar process (1), translucency with fluid level (2), in the synovial cavity. Picture taken in upright position.

A translucency with a fluid level must always bring to mind an intraarticular fracture. The fracture causes release of blood as well as marrow fat into the synovial fluid. The fatty material floats on top and is more radiotranslucent than watery fluid. Hence the typical radiographic picture which in this case draws attention to an avulsion fracture of the tibial attachment of the anterior cruciate ligament. In cases of trauma to the knee it is advisable to take pictures in different positions including standing, to detect the presence of lipohaemarthrosis.

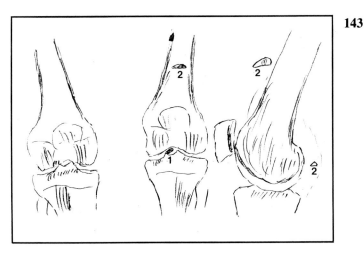

143

144 March (stress) fracture – osteomalacia

Pseudofracture (1), callus formation (2).

March fracture occurs commonly in soldiers and affects particularly the 2nd and 3rd metatarsals. Sometimes a march fracture cannot be demonstrated on radiography at the onset of symptoms (pain after marching and local swelling) and only comes to light when callus is produced. After a march, stress fractures can also occur in the fibula, femur and ischiopubic rami.

The same sites can also be affected in osteomalacia. Osteomalacia is the result of a disorder of Vitamin D metabolism which can occur as a result of various conditions, for instance a lack of sunlight, nutritional disorders, malabsorption, liver and kidney malfunction.

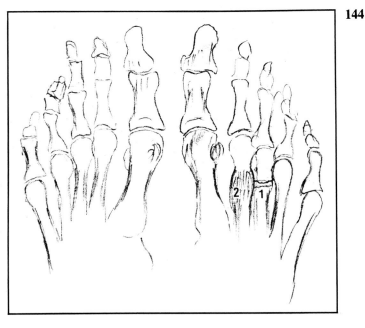

144

145

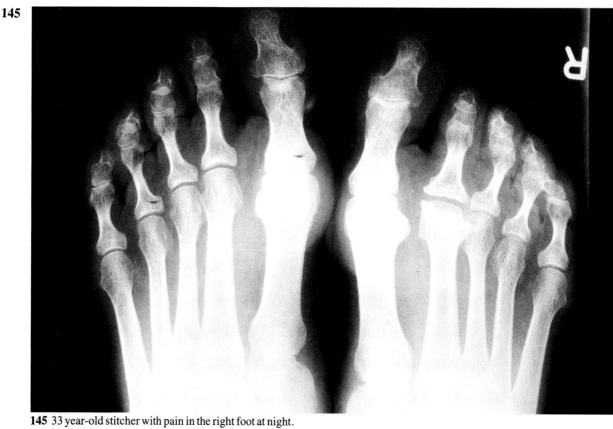

145 33 year-old stitcher with pain in the right foot at night.

146

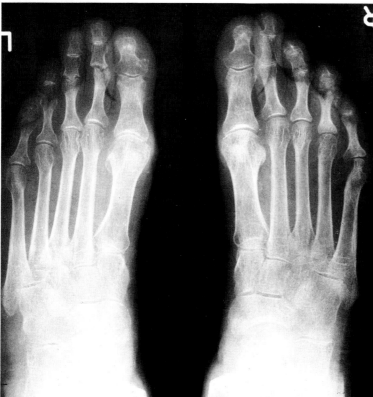

146 37 year-old housewife who has suffered from polyarthritis since the age of 7, has responded well to treatment with gold salts, now requests supporting soles. There is a past history of psoriasis.

145 Freiberg's osteochondrosis

Flattening and expansion of the head of the second right metatarsal and base of the proximal phalanx of the same toe (arrows).

Osteonecrosis of the head of the second metatarsal is one of the commonest sites of aseptic necrosis of bone. It is a lesion which develops during the growth phase and is almost always symptomless. Owing to the disturbance of anatomical equilibrium, secondary arthrosis and hypertrophic osteophytosis may later develop and lead to metatarsalgia. Reassurance regarding the cause of the discomfort usually suffices, sometimes a support is prescribed which will relieve the pressure of weight bearing.

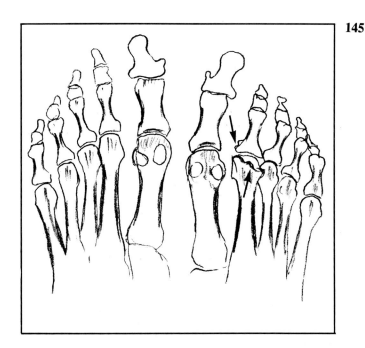

145

146 Psoriatic polyarthritis

Diminution of joint space (1), erosions (2), joint destruction with bone resorption (3).

It requires a special technique and experience to discover erosions on a radiograph of the feet. Left and right joints need to be compared methodically. Here one finds that the head of the right fifth metatarsal is eroded both medially and laterally; that the head of the third left metatarsal shows erosion where it contacts the head of the second metatarsal, and that the second and third left proximal interphalangeal joints are affected.

It is often difficult to evaluate the interphalangeal joints on radiography of the feet since they are usually in a position of flexion and therefore do not show up well.

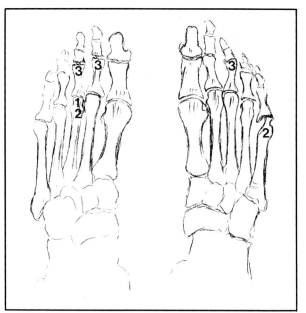

146

147

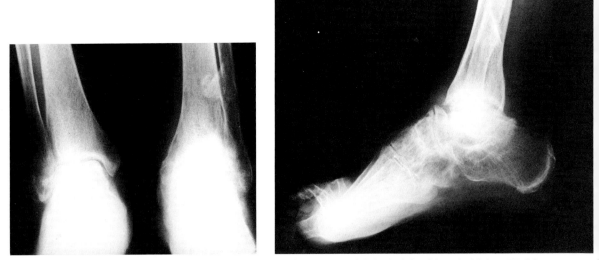

147 56 year-old miner's wife with stiff joints for many years and now pain mainly in the left ankle and mid-foot. Walking on uneven ground is particularly difficult. A while ago she fell and hurt her leg.

148

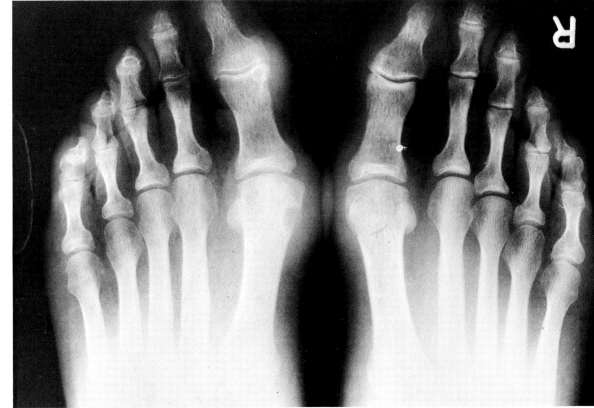

148 60 year-old baker complaining of 3 painful attacks per year in the foot and sometimes the knee over a period of 10 years.

147 Rheumatoid arthritis – secondary arthrosis

Diminution of joint space (1), subchondral sclerosis (2), fracture line (3) with slight displacement, callus formation; mid-foot or intertarsal arthritis (4) with secondary osteophyte formation (5), metatarsophalangeal subluxations (6).

The intertarsal joints are more frequently affected by rheumatoid arthritis than the ankle.

After the arrest of active arthritis, spontaneous or through medication, there often remains an irreversible loss of cartilage which leads to secondary arthrosis with sclerosis and osteophytosis particularly in weight bearing areas. At this stage powerful short or long acting antiphlogistics which in themselves may be dangerous, are not indicated and one should resort to conservative measures or else decide on surgical intervention.

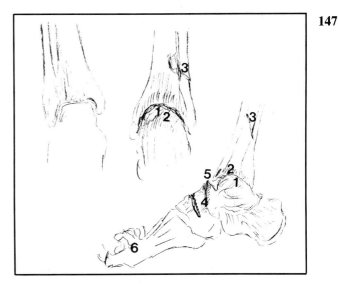

147

148 Gouty arthritis

Paraarticular geode (1), soft tissue swelling (tophus) (2), early erosions (3).

In cases of advanced gout the radiological picture consists of diminution of joint space, marginal osteophytosis, geodes or punched-out translucencies near the bone extremities. Any of these may be absent or occur alone. A geode is the only typical sign although it is not pathognomonic, since it may also occur in rheumatoid arthritis and in arthrosis.
Geodes occur mainly in the hands and feet particularly if there are urate deposits in the vicinity. Geodes are round or oval with a diameter of a few millimetres to one centimetre. The margins are clearly demarcated as though they have been punched out. Some geodes are subchondrally or laterally situated.

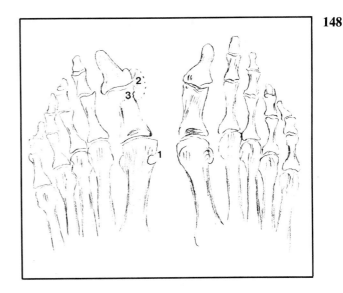

148

149

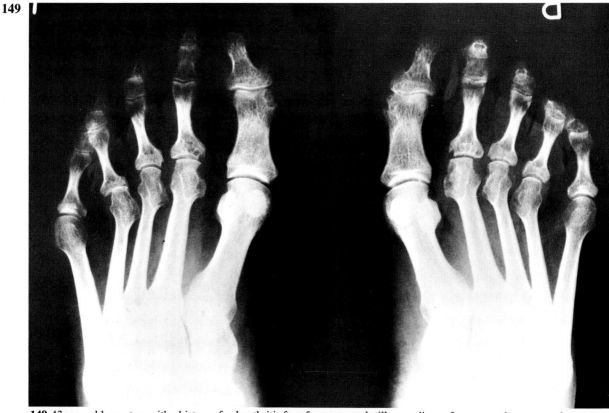

149 43 year-old secretary with a history of polyarthritis for a few years and still some discomfort on wearing narrow shoes.

150

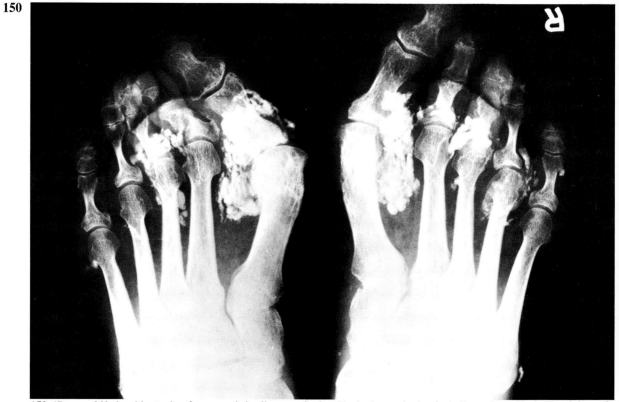

150 47 year-old lady with attacks of severe pain in elbows and soles. Has had an operation for hallux valgus. She has hard, irregular subcutaneous nodules.

149 Rheumatoid arthritis

Narrowing of joint space (1), erosions (2) with sharply defined edges, subchondral cystic translucencies (3).

In rheumatoid arthritis there are radiological signs which indicate the degree of activity of the lesions. When the erosions are sharply outlined or have sclerotic margins, the local inflammatory reactions are quiescent and only the scars are left. It is important to recognise these signs as they may determine future treatment.

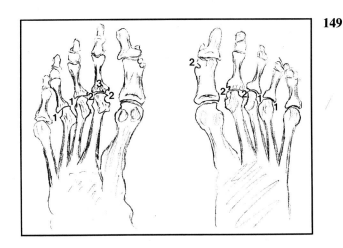

150 Systemic sclerosis – Thibierge-Weissenbach syndrome

Calcifications in the paraarticular soft tissues (1), signs of bone resection (2), hallux valgus (3), bone resorption (4) proximal phalanx left second toe.

The occurrence of paraarticular calcifications in the soft tissues of the hands, elbows and feet is called the Thibierge-Weissenbach syndrome. Actually the calcifications represent only part of a more widely distributed connective tissue disorder namely systemic sclerosis, with sclerosis of the skin and telangiectasis, pulmonary fibrosis, sclerosis of the esophagus and small bowel. These signs are grouped together in the term C.R.E.S.T. syndrome: C for calcinosis, R for Raynaud's phenomenon, E for esophagus, S for systemic sclerosis, T for telangiectasis.

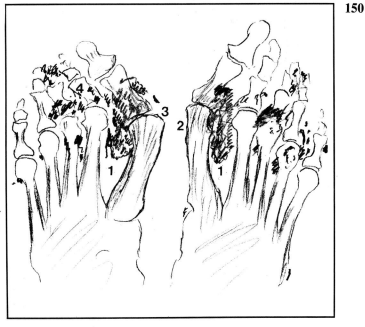

151

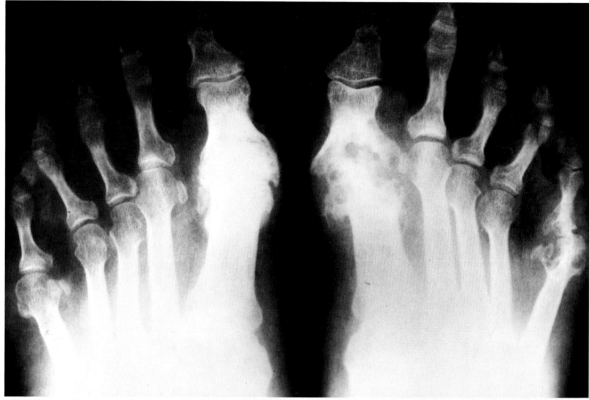

151 68 year-old brewer under observation for liver trouble. History of recurring arthritis for 30 years, especially in the feet. At the moment no pains in the feet.

152

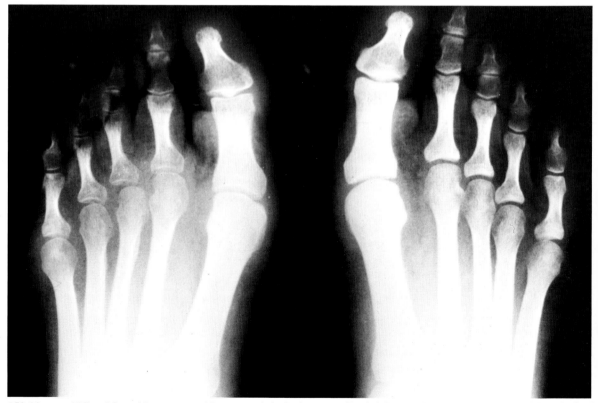

152 23 year-old Spanish working woman with severe pain in the fore part of her left foot and less marked pain in the right wrist for 5 months. No rheumatoid arthritis factor found in the serum.

151 Gouty arthritis

Joint destruction with hypertrophic bone reaction (1) and geodes (2).

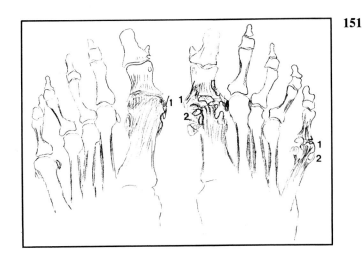

Radiologically gouty arthritis is distinguished from rheumatoid arthritis by its hypertrophic bone reaction with obvious osteophytosis. The erosions are generally larger than those of rheumatoid arthritis hence we talk of geodes. The geodes are often further away from the synovial reflexion than in rheumatoid arthritis.

Despite the striking radiological abnormalities, usually monoarticular, sufferers from gout maintain very good function outside the acute attacks.

152 Seronegative oligoarthritis

Periarticular osteoporosis (1), periosteal reaction (2).

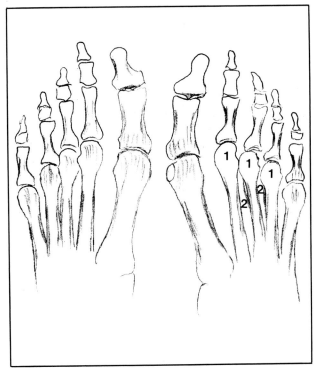

An oligoarthritis lasting more than 4 months, yielding a negative reaction for rheumatoid arthritis factor on serological examination and to which no other definite diagnostic label can be attached, is best classified as a seronegative oligopolyarthritis. It is now known that a fair number of syndromes associated with the presence of HLA B27 antigen can start as an oligoarthritis. After months or years, other facets of the syndrome come to light such as spondylitis, sacroiliitis, uveitis, enteritis, erythema nodosum, psoriasis, urethritis. By virtue of the combination of signs one can then diagnose Reiter's syndrome, Bechterew's disease or ankylosing spondylitis, psoriatic arthritis, arthritis with erythema nodosum or with ulcerative colitis or Crohn's disease.

Since these patients with a seronegative oligoarthritis have a better prognosis with virtually no residual disability, it is important to distinguish them from those who suffer from an arthritis associated with the presence of rheumatoid arthritis factor in the serum.

153

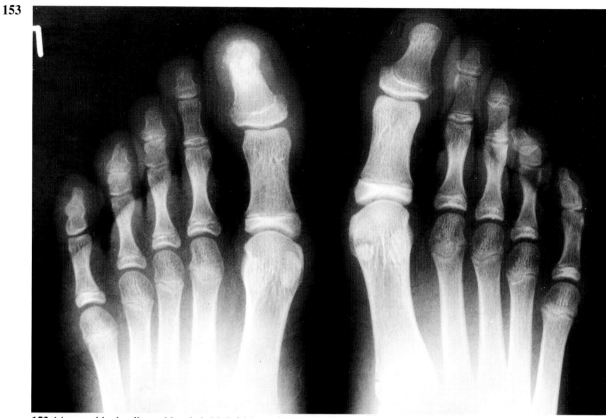

153 14 year-old schoolboy with pain in his left big toe for 3 years, for which footbaths were given.

154

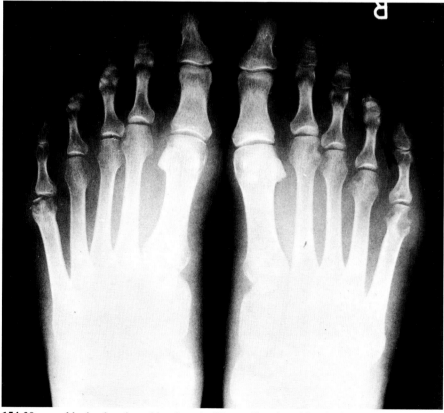

154 30 year-old schoolteacher with pain and stiffness of hands and feet for 1 year.

153 Osteomyelitis

Sclerosis (1) of left big toe distal phalanx with sequestrum (2).

In the early stages osteomyelitis presents no radiological signs. Osteomyelitis usually affects a single bone, frequently the tibial or femoral shaft. After a few weeks local resorption with osteoporosis becomes evident. Some parts of the bone undergo necrosis due to compression of bloodvessels, and are not resorbed because of the presence of pus; these circumstances lead to sequestrum formation. Periosteum in the vicinity will react after a few weeks and this can be seen on radiography. After years pus and some sequestra may be evacuated through the skin with formation of fistulae.

Osteomyelitis occurs most commonly in adolescents. In old age the disease may flare up again.

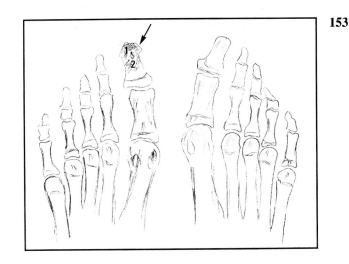

153

154 Rheumatoid arthritis

Erosion of the head of the fifth metatarsal in both feet (arrows).

Radiological signs of rheumatoid arthritis affecting the feet usually manifest many months after the onset of complaints. Erosions affect above all the lateral side of the head of the fifth metatarsal. It may be possible to discover erosions before the patient complains of pain in this region. Besides the metatarsophalangeal joint of the fifth toe, that of the second and also of the third can frequently be affected.

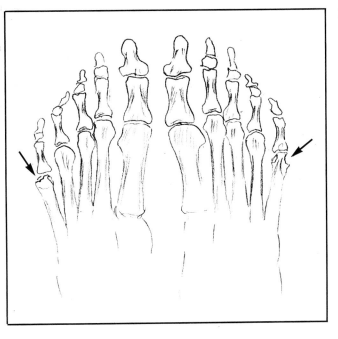

154

155

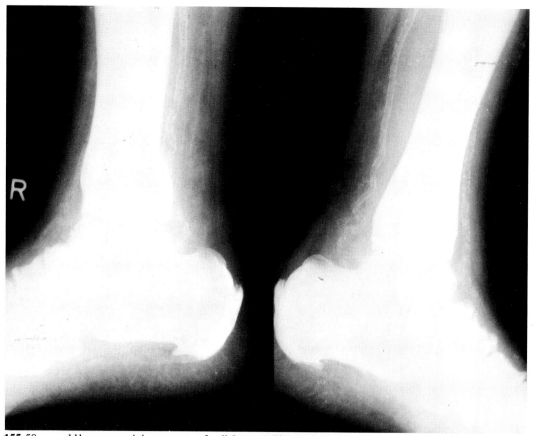

155 58 year-old brewer receiving treatment for diabetes mellitus and psoriasis. Has regular attacks of pain in the heel.

156

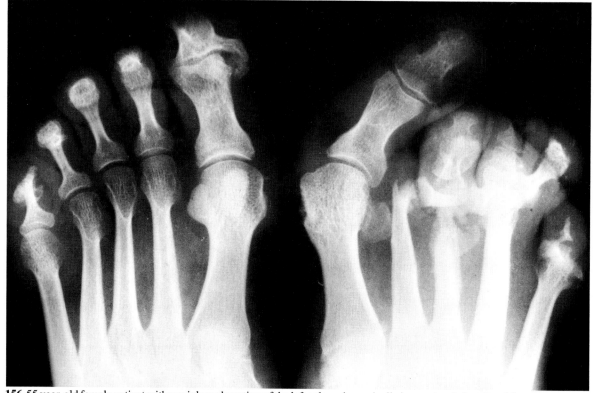

156 55 year-old female patient with a painless ulceration of the left sole and a gradually increasing deformity of the toes.

155 Enthesopathy – achilles tendinitis – calcaneal spur

Enthesopathy (1), calcaneal spur (2), osteophytosis (3), arterial calcification (4).

Pain in the heel can be caused by an Achilles tendinitis or a bursitis associated with a calcaneal spur.

The Achilles tendinitis may present radiological signs of erosion of the back of the calcaneus or calcification at the insertion of the tendon or both. A calcaneal spur is an exostosis on the traction epiphysis of the plantar aponeurosis. Bursitis in the region of the spur produces pain on walking. Many people have a calcaneal spur without pain. Surgical intervention is rarely indicated. Tendinitis at the calcaneus is common in athletes but may also occur in Reiter's syndrome, ankylosing spondylitis and psoriatic spondylarthropathy.

Enthesopathy and tendinitis occur also in metabolic (diabetes) and storage (xanthomatosis) diseases.

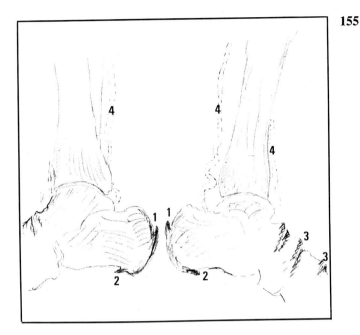

155

156 Mutilating acropathy – neuroarthropathy

Resorption of phalanges (1), and metatarsals (2), erosions (3), joint destruction (4), hypertrophic bone reaction (5), periostitis (6).

Neuropathy of the peripheral sensory nerves can give rise to destructive lesions not only of bone but also of the skin which results in a perforating ulcer. A similar neuropathy and its sequelae can occur in leprosy, poisoning, syphilis and as a hereditary familial disease, Thévenard's disease.

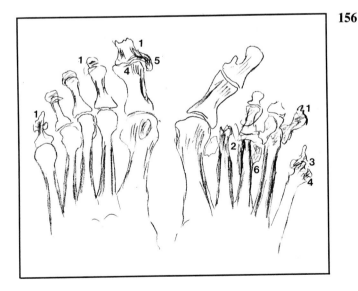

156

157

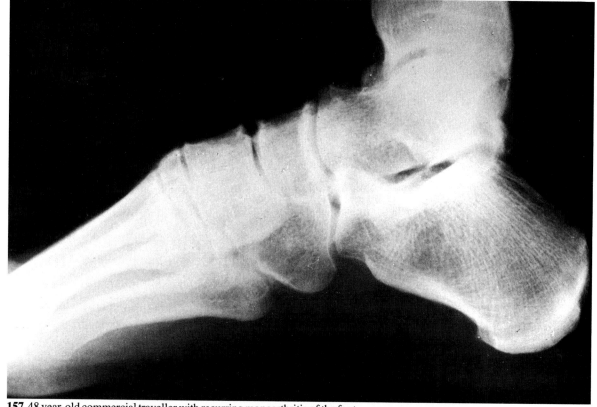

157 48 year-old commercial traveller with recurring monoarthritis of the foot.

158

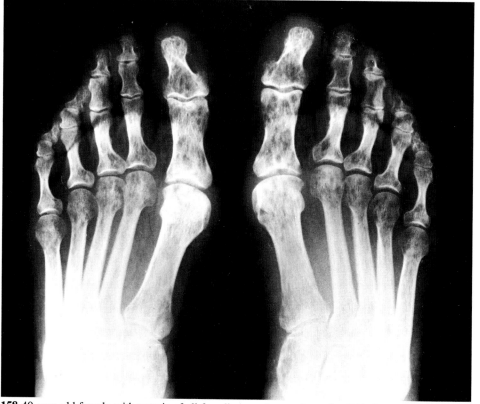

158 40 year-old female with paresis of all four limbs, a hypercalcaemia of 11.5 per cent and kidney stones. The neurologist suggested Guillain-Barré syndrome.

157 Gouty arthritis

Osteophytosis of the mid-foot joints producing a 'pied hérissé' (arrows).

Although gout so often attacks the big toe metatarsophalangeal joint, arthritis of the mid-foot joints also occurs frequently. Repeated attacks of these intertarsal joints leads to typical radiological signs of joint space narrowing and formation of multiple osteophytes along the dorsum of the foot which gives a spiky appearance resembling the back of a hedgehog, hence the French term.

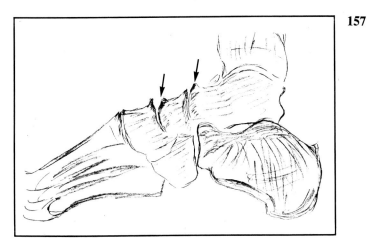

157

158 Immobilisation osteoporosis

Mottled appearance from patchy osteoporosis (1).

Immobilisation, without regard to its cause, produces serious decalcification which presents the typical radiological picture of diffuse patchy translucency. When the immobilisation involves a large part of the skeleton, hypercalcaemia and hypercalciuria may ensue with the formation of kidney stones.

A similar immobilisation osteoporosis is seen in algoneurodystrophy (Südeck-Reflex dystrophy) where there is no absolute immobilisation.

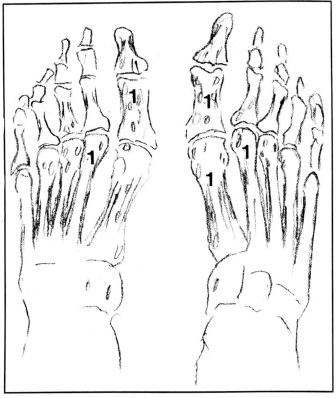

158

159

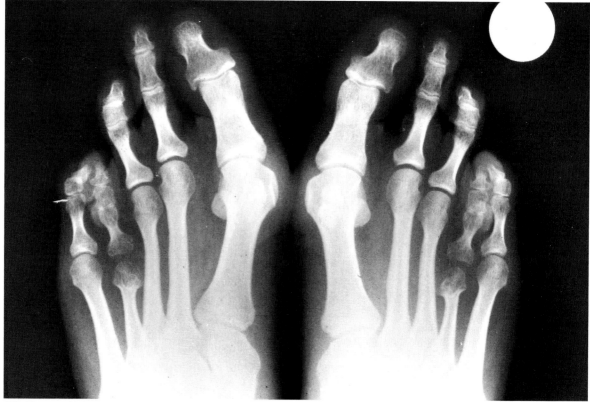

159 30 year-old housewife admitted because of synovitis of the hands and feet, and a positive LE phenomenon. Congenital shortening of the 4th toe.

160

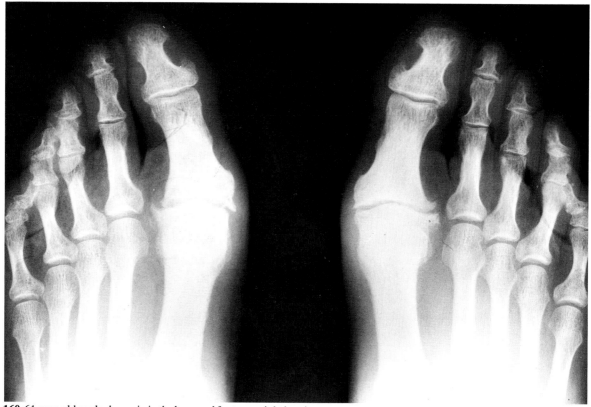

160 61 year-old gaoler has pain in the knee and foot on weight bearing.

159 Brachymetatarsia

Shortening of the metatarsal (1) and proximal phalanx (2) of the 4th toe.

Like brachymetacarpia, brachymetatarsia can be an expression of an underlying congenital defect involving other organs such as the ovary (Turner's syndrome) and ('pseudo') pseudohypoparathyroidism where there is an altered sensitivity to parathormone.

Brachymetatarsia can equally be an isolated phenomenon and have nothing to do with the complaint of the patient, as in this case.

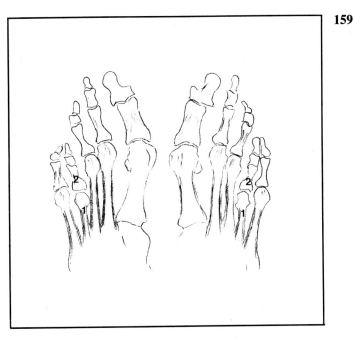

159

160 Hallux valgus plus arthrosis of the big toe metatarsophalangeal joint

Uneven joint space diminution (1), marginal osteophytosis (2), sclerosis (3).

Hallux valgus and arthrosis of the big toe usually occur bilaterally. They are often associated with arthrosis of the small joints of the hands, particularly the distal interphalangeal joints where Heberden's nodes may occur.

A hallux valgus may appear during adolescence but usually expresses itself fully in adulthood. It usually produces a mechanical hindrance in the shoe and can become a stiff toe, hallux rigidus. A bursa which often develops between the skin and the osteophyte may become inflamed.

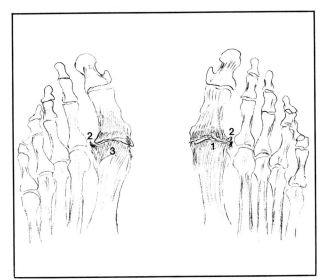

160

Index

All numbers refer to the cases described in the book and *not* to pages